Listening as Work in Primary Care

Simon Cocksedge

Foreword by

Martin Roland

Epilogue by

Carl May

Radcliffe Publishing
Oxford • Seattle

Radcliffe Publishing Ltd
18 Marcham Road
Abingdon
Oxon OX14 1AA
United Kingdom

www.radcliffe-oxford.com
Electronic catalogue and worldwide online ordering facility.

British Library Cataloguing in Publication Data

A catalogue record for this book is available from the British Library.

ISBN 1 85775 636 3

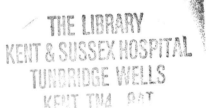
Typeset by Aarontype Ltd, Easton, Bristol
Printed and bound by TJ International Ltd, Padstow, Cornwall

Contents

Foreword   v

Preface   vi

Acknowledgements   x

About the author   xi

How to use this book   xii

Introduction   1

Section 1   Choices in listening   15

1   The importance of listening   17

2   Choosing to listen   29

3   Choosing not to listen   35

Section 2   Listening work and relationships   47

4   Cumulative listening and relationships   49

5   Pastoral work in primary care   59

6   Holding work: description   67

7   Holding work: discussion   79

Section 3   Boundaries and self in listening work   93

8   Listening work and organisational boundaries   95

9   Listening work and interpersonal boundaries   105

10   Work and self: boundaries   115

11   Work and self: adequacy and sincerity   123

12   Listening as work in primary care   131

Postscript: 'I just listened'   155

Epilogue   159

Appendix I   Methodology   161

Appendix II   Communication skills   162

Appendix III   Further reading   169

Index   171

Foreword

At a time when GPs are concentrating as never before on bio-medical aspects of their work, this book is a very timely reminder of the importance of inter-personal aspects of the care that we provide for patients. The motto of the Royal College of General Practitioners is *Cum Scientia Caritas* which emphasises that general practice must combine scientific knowledge with caring. This book reminds us of the legitimacy of one of the key aspects of general practice.

Simon Cocksedge describes listening to patients as an important and valid part of the work that we do as GPs. For me, the most telling quotation in the book was from a GP registrar who said 'I didn't do any medicine – I just listened.' Simon argues that listening is work, and he describes the choices that we have during consultations to allow patients to express their problems, the importance of listening to the development of long term relationships with patients, and the importance of 'being with' patients during significant life experiences.

While GPs now have many incentives to provide high quality clinical care, Simon describes the barriers which exist to providing high quality inter-personal care. These include the pressures of time and the need that we feel to protect ourselves from some of the emotional aspects of our work. This book is a most important reminder of the need for GPs to preserve a balance between the various aspects of their work. The GP registrar quoted above is wrong. Listening is legitimate work.

Martin Roland
Director
National Primary Care Research and Development Centre
April 2005

Preface

This book has arisen from reflections on patients' everyday stories in my work as a general practitioner (GP) in Derbyshire. I have been a GP principal in a semi-rural practice with some 8300 patients served by a full primary care team since 1986. Over several years, I reflected on the mandate that GPs are given by society to listen and to be available if required. I also considered boundaries in my relationships with patients arising from specific instances and encounters.

My first reflections explored GPs' listening within the consultation, and the skills required:

> An 18-year-old came to see me in surgery today with abdominal bloating and a missed period. I used simple listening skills (open questions, reflecting, pausing, summarising, body language and so forth) to hear her story, which came tumbling out, and to make a plan. It was the last appointment on Friday afternoon so she did not receive any more than that and a follow-up the next week.

Sometimes a period of listening, separate to the initial presenting problem, is needed within a consultation:

> A 65-year-old man, whom I know well, came in with a pre-operation form. Having signed this, I listened for five or ten minutes while he discussed general anaesthetics, his fears of death and of not waking up from the anaesthetic.

> A young woman came in with a cold. We ended up exploring the fact that her termination was some seven months ago and the baby would be due today if she had kept the pregnancy: 'All my friends are having babies ... I feel so empty – you should feel nine months full and yet you're empty.'

GPs will recognise these scenarios. But do they feel comfortable or competent undertaking such listening, and do they see it as their role? Some people attend their GP without any overt medical problem:

> She is in her thirties, single after the break-up of her long-term relationship some two years ago. I have treated her for depression a couple of times

since then: 'What does it all mean, Simon? Why is it like this? Why can't I just be happy?'. We grapple with the issues. She seems to be searching, deeply.

Such grappling with issues and life events, more pastoral than clinical, occurs regularly in the GP surgery, but what do GPs feel about such work?

Some patients seem to need to touch base with their GP regularly:

Mrs A is chronically depressed. She has been on antidepressants for several years and has severe relationship and financial problems. We have an agreement that she will come and see me every two months for a routine consultation and she is there, every eight weeks, without fail. I listen, she tells me the same tales with variations, I give her her medication and she departs: 'Thank you doctor, I don't know what I'd do without you, you keep me going.'

Others attend regularly for a while and then their needs change. Some have an agreement, with others it just 'happens'. A small but significant routine task for many GPs, involving seeing a patient regularly for ongoing support over a period of time.

The pressures on the individual GP are often considerable. At any one time, I am aware that I have some patients who are at the front of my mind for a variety of reasons:

Mrs N is in her mid-eighties and has struggled to cope alone since her husband died two years ago. She suffers from severe osteo-arthritis and congestive cardiac failure, both of which restrict her to an armchair most of the time. Social services and our nurses visit two or three times a day but despite this, she is deteriorating gently.

How long will she manage at home? Her son, who lives away, telephones me several times and I visit regularly as the situation progresses. We are both concerned for her.

I have known Mr and Mrs F for some years and we meet at occasional social occasions. Mr F and I see each other regularly on the committee of a local club. He telephones me at home on a Sunday morning, worried that Mrs F has had a stroke. I feel torn as I am not on duty and am busy with our family. Nevertheless, I visit and manage the situation.

It is often such patients who are pushing me to my limits, creating pressures in my daily work which require managing. They also touch on the boundaries

I draw around work and the rest of my life. They may cause me to reflect on aspects of myself, such as awareness of my adequacy (or not) both as a GP and as a person.

Three areas of questioning emerged from my reflections on these stories of everyday work as a family doctor, and these have formed the basis for this book:

- How do GPs conceptualise listening work in their encounters with patients?
- How do GPs manage the effects of this work over time, the cumulative listening that builds relationships?
- In everyday general practice, how do doctors frame the limits to their listening, both with their patients and for themselves?

I investigated these questions by listening to the stories told by experienced general practitioners about their perceptions of their everyday work with patients. Although I have used qualitative methods (described in Appendix I) developed in the field of sociology, this is an investigation of primary care written by a practising GP. It offers insights into the everyday work and world of a group of GPs in one area of England, and reflects the nature of general practice at the beginning of the twenty-first century. The field of study is the everyday business of being a family doctor and the inter- and intra-personal phenomena that arise as a result. There is no intention to contribute directly to wider debates about healthcare policy, clinical govern-ance or clinical effectiveness. Perhaps this is because, although such issues may form a structure within which GPs work, they perceive that the true centre of their everyday work remains each patient who comes through the consulting room door.

Terminology

In order to use consistent terminology throughout this book, I have used the following definitions.

- *Interaction* – a single encounter between doctor and patient, either within a consultation or in another setting (for example, by telephone, in a social setting).
- *Relationship* – the ongoing cumulative result of a series of interactions between doctor and patient.

- *Encounter* – collective term for both individual interactions and ongoing relationships between doctors and patients.

Throughout the book, when a doctor's name appears by a quote, it is not their true name. Any reference in the text to 'these doctors' means the GPs who took part in the original study on which this book is based.

Simon Cocksedge
April 2005

Acknowledgements

This book could not have been written without the help of a great many people, to all of whom I give my thanks.

First among them must be two Carls from the Division of Primary Care at the University of Manchester. Professor Carl Whitehouse has advised on this project since my first ideas landed on his desk. He suggested that I talk to Carl May (now Professor of Medical Sociology at the University of Newcastle). This second Carl has helped me to develop those initial ideas, supervised my work, and has been consistently supportive and helpful throughout the lifespan of this project. I am very grateful to them both.

The bulk of the fieldwork took place during a sabbatical in 1999. Thanks to my partners at Thornbrook Surgery for their support in allowing me the time, to the National Health Service for funding my prolonged study leave, and to the National Primary Care Research and Development Centre for funding additional protected study time. The backbone of this work is some 35 hours of interviews with GPs, who all gave generously of their time and views. I am indebted to them all, as I am to Alison Burgess, Caroline Connolly and Denise Mukadam for secretarial and transcribing support at the Rusholme Academic Unit. Thanks also to those at the University of Manchester and elsewhere who have contributed, knowingly or unknowingly, to this work at various stages. I am particularly grateful to Peter Bower, Chris Dowrick, Nicola Mead, David Riddell, Anne Rogers, Martin Roland, Nicholas Sagovsky, Keith Sharp and Val Wass.

My last and biggest thanks are to two groups from whom I have learnt, and from whom I continue to learn, so much. These are, first, the people of the High Peak in Derbyshire and, second, my family without whose continuing loving support this work would not have seen the light of day.

How to use this book

The aim of this book is to encourage health professionals in primary care to reflect on listening in their work with patients – the choices they make, the relationships which emerge and the boundaries or limits that they put in place. Although the book is based on a study of doctors in primary care, the lessons about listening could equally apply to others in caring professions.

The Preface briefly presents the emergence of this book from my experience as a GP. The Introduction places this work in the context of relevant primary care literature – it is quite long and should be ignored by readers to whom theoretical arguments do not appeal! The three sections that follow focus on listening, relationships and the boundaries or limits doctors establish around their work and themselves. Lastly, Chapter 12 and the Postscript draw some conclusions and raise some questions for the future of primary care and listening work. The caveat about the Introduction also applies to the second half of Chapter 12.

I hope that this book will be helpful to doctors in training for work in primary care, and to established GPs. However, this is *not* a textbook of communication or listening skills. I have outlined some of these skills in Appendix II and, in Appendix III, I have made some suggestions for further reading that doctors in training might find helpful to use alongside this book.

About the author

Simon Cocksedge is a general practitioner in Chapel-en-le-Frith, High Peak, Derbyshire. He is a lecturer in primary care and communication at the University of Manchester, and scheme organiser for general practice vocational training in Macclesfield.

For
Sally, Matt, Sam and Chaz,
and the people of the High Peak,
from whom I learn so much

Introduction

This introduction provides a theoretical background and context for the work presented in the remaining chapters and is in three sections. First, I consider the place of stories about primary care, such as those outlined in the Preface and the accounts on which this book is based. Alongside their intrinsic interest, they offer a narrative window on what actually happens in general practice and in general practitioners' encounters with their patients. Clearly, such windows have limitations, but that does not make the view they provide any less valid.

Second, I present a trend in the literature from 'bedside to biomedical', from a personal model of illness to a hospital and laboratory model. I then suggest that this has parallels in the study of the doctor–patient encounter, from a longer-term relational context to a more specific analysis of behaviours, skills and tasks in the interaction.

Third, with particular reference to patient-centred medicine, I discuss tensions between the ideals of doctors in primary care and the practical application of these ideals in everyday practice.

The importance of stories

There was a time when the only tools at the doctor's disposal were a full and careful hearing of the patient's story, a cursory examination, followed by application of largely ineffective treatments. Then came understanding of clinical examination, with the ability to tease out clinical signs as clues to diagnosis. The increasing availability of investigations and treatments reduces reliance on the history as a diagnostic or therapeutic manoeuvre. As a result, it has been suggested that the patient's story may matter less than used to be the case.[1] In contrast, the recent interest in narrative in medicine[2–4] has been perhaps a reaction both to these trends and to the increasing emphasis on evidence-based medicine. The latter, it has been suggested, 'can imply a simplistic and mechanistic world-view in which cause and effect are easily distinguished':[5]

> The art of medicine is founded upon context, anecdote, patient stories of illness, and personal experience; these are classified as 'lower quality' in the

hierarchy of evidence, but have an equally valid contribution to decision making. ... It is this integration of 'stories', anecdotes, case histories, and evidence that is one of the successes of primary care. A positive approach could be to put the flesh of clinical stories, case histories, qualitative research, and other rich sources of information onto the hard bones of Evidence Based Medicine.[5]

Integration of sources of data is the key. Medicine has been described as 'fundamentally narrative',[2] and narrative has been used by doctors for a long time in the form of anecdotes[6] or stories.[7] Such stories may be:

> ... stories told by patients to doctors (symptoms), by doctors to doctors (case histories) and by doctors to patients (explanations); stories told about doctors and patients (medicine in literature — both as truth and metaphor); stories told by doctors to their students (anecdotal teaching).[1]

This has parallels with the place of story telling in society:

> Story telling has always played a central role in human culture. From the earliest recorded history people have interacted through the exchange of stories as a means of entertainment, recording history and conveying a moral code. Narratives (myths) have been the first cognitive and linguistic tools by which people have tried to achieve a sense of coherence and personal understanding. They are suited for making sense of one's own life in time. They have also been instrumental in providing the social and cultural codes which went into the construction of societies. Stories can therefore be considered ordering mechanisms both on the intra-personal and the inter-personal level.[8]

Stories involving general practitioners (GPs) can be subdivided into stories *by* GPs and stories *about* GPs. Stories about GPs may be fictional or non-fictional. Fiction allows insight into contemporary popular culture and myths about the medical profession. An example from general practice would be *The Citadel*.[9] Non-fictional stories about GPs abound in the literature, some descriptive,[10] some more idealised,[11] some in-depth and autobiographical,[12] and some used analytically to explore the clinical encounter.[13]

Similarly, stories by GPs about their work can range from practical or political outlines[14] to more idealised reminiscences[15] via accounts of everyday practice.[16] Perhaps more intimate, and at a different level, are stories by GPs that give clues both to the narrative content of the individual GP–patient interaction,[17] to the socio-cultural context in which they work[18] and to the ongoing narrative of the GP–patient relationship over the years.[19] Poetry by GPs adds other glimpses into the doctor–patient encounter and the work of the GP.[20]

> In contemporary literary criticism and in the theory of human sciences, narrative is understood as a way of knowing.[2]

The narrative stories by doctors on which this book is based provide insights into the taken-for-granted, everyday world and work of medicine and the GP, both the public 'front region' and the more private 'back region'.[21] These insights are complementary to, and may be integrated with, the 'hard bones of Evidence Based Medicine'.[5] Such integration of data sources offers the key to fuller understanding.

Bedside to biomedical

The start of the National Health Service (NHS) in 1948 formally established primary (community) and secondary (hospital) care, for which there was no direct charge. The subsequent development of general medical practice through the Porritt[22] and Gillie[23] reports firmly established the GP as the first point of contact for healthcare in the UK, with general practice as a specialty in its own right. Around the same time, during the middle decades of the twentieth century, doctors, who had previously 'felt so helpless to do anything' in the face of advanced organic disease,[24] acquired therapeutic tools which transformed the practice of medicine and influenced their relationship with their patients. Treatments started to become widely available, such as antibiotics, insulin and liver extract for pernicious anaemia. Nicholls, in describing his grandfather's general practice at the end of the nineteenth century, noted:

> When there was little or nothing that could be done to cure infectious diseases, the personal approach may have been more important than it is today. Charm, kindness and good manners were a necessity for high success and some of the practitioners of old had these in abundance.[25]

Previously, the sick had selected their practitioners using their own assessment of the moral integrity and professional skill of the practitioner, and thus the 'interaction was joined on the basis of personal empathy between the parties'.[26] For the doctor, directly dependent upon the patient for his income and with few adequate therapies, a good bedside manner was crucial. Gibson wrote from his own experience:

The coming of penicillin and the other antibiotics had in themselves brought about a subtle and dramatic change in the general practitioner's life. Perhaps the most significant change, and one not fully appreciated at the time, was that in a certain respect they came between doctor and patient and so, inevitably, changed the doctor patient relationship. There was no longer need to visit two or three times a day or to make lengthy visits. Capsules left on the bedside table, to be taken two at a time every six hours, reduced the visits to one a day, if that, and the length of the illness from weeks to days.[14]

Hence, changes in society and in technology impinged on the doctor–patient relationship. The encounter was no longer that of client and professional, organised around payment of a fee, because doctors became public servants. The development of effective treatments enabled doctors to significantly alter the course of disease and to prolong life expectancy. The bedside medicine model of the late eighteenth century, in which illness was largely understood by both doctor and patient through the narrative of the patient,[27] was superseded by a biomedical hospital and laboratory model. This has been called a shift from a person-orientated to an object-orientated cosmology of illness,[26] or a swing 'from *illness* as a subjective (and individualised) experience, towards *disease* as objective (and generalised) phenomena. ... Medicine shifted from the bedside to the hospital'.[28]

These societal, technological and relational changes have not only influenced the practice of medicine, but are also reflected in the way that academics investigate the GP–patient interaction. The shift from a bedside model of illness to a biomedical hospital and laboratory model has parallels with the shift from the study of relationship in the doctor–patient encounter to a more technical, quantificatory and skill-based approach.

The emergence of general practice as a separate academic discipline within the profession of medicine (the Royal College of General Practitioners was founded in 1952) was facilitated in part by taking a biographical approach to studying doctor–patient interactions. This was achieved by emphasising the importance of social and psychological factors (alongside the biological factors that remained largely the province of the hospital-based doctor),[29] and by focusing on the consultation as potentially therapeutic in its own right:[28,30]

The conduct of doctor–patient interaction ... became central to the doctrine of general practice, because it offered an important *theoretical* basis for a kind of medicine that lacked complex diagnostic and treatment technologies at a time when technological expansionism marked out the more general terrain of medicine.[31]

Highly influential in these developments was the psychotherapist Michael Balint. In the 1950s, not long after the formation of the NHS and at a time when general practice was somewhat in the doldrums, he set up group work for a small number of GPs. Balint acted as the group facilitator, and out of these experiences came his book, *The Doctor, His Patient and the Illness* (first edition 1957, second edition 1963; I have used the latter in this book).[30] GPs were observed, through their contributions to the group, discussing their daily work over two to three years, allowing continuity and follow-up of individual patients.

One aim of this research was 'a reasonably thorough examination of the ever-changing doctor–patient relationship, i.e. the study of the pharmacology of the drug "doctor"'.[30] Key messages concerned listening (seen as a new skill, very different to medical history taking), the 'mutual investment company' that forms the 'long and often intimate connection' between patient and GP, the doctor's own emotional reactions to such listening and relating, and the different roles that may be required of the GP (for example, diagnostician, obstetrician, listener, friend of the family). For the first time, GP–patient interaction was thought of both as suitable for study and as therapeutic in its own right. This was a major change and started GPs on a process of reflection about their everyday work, their relationships to their patients, their overall role and their skills in communicating.

In *The Doctor–Patient Relationship*, Browne and Freeling[32] reflected on cases from their own work as GPs, and on 'experience and the hard facts of life'. They assumed an ongoing nature for GPs' relationships with their patients and differentiated three characteristics of the GP not shared by hospital specialists.

- The GP is 'the doctor who has first contact with the patient (and so) he must practise in other than ideal circumstances'.
- The GP 'does not limit the type of illness which the patient may present to him … and must call upon specialist help in diagnosis and treatment. His achievement must rest on being an adequate doctor to each and every patient … accepting this responsibility and the frustrating inability to be perfect'.
- Many GPs have long-term, ongoing, sometimes 'lifelong' relationships with their patients.[32]

The subjective, personal and case-based work of Browne and Freeling contrasts with the more behavioural, task-focused research of Byrne and Long[33] in *Doctors Talking to Patients: a study of the verbal behaviour of general practitioners consulting in their surgeries*. This was significant because, for the first time, it provided a 'study of the behaviours of doctors in their surgeries … Its purpose is to provide a non-judgemental view of how they behave'.[33] The researchers were 'seeking to discover what patterns of behaviour doctors appeared to follow in their consulting rooms and the degree to which the patterns were repetitive'.[33] From more than 2500 audiotapes of consultations, Byrne and Long defined a logical sequence of events within consultations and were able to establish styles of consulting (doctor centred or patient centred). Byrne went on to analyse non-verbal behaviour in real consultations using video recording to freeze and recapture important words or pauses so that they could be studied.[34] This innovatory work has had a strong influence on the study of the doctor–patient relationship and the development of training for GPs. For the first time, the interaction was analysed in terms of *behaviours*. Many subsequent studies have also emphasised the behavioural aspects of the interaction, in part because these are measurable and easily teachable, at the expense of the study of *relationships* and the person of the doctor in GP–patient interactions.

For example, nearly a decade later, in *The Consultation: an approach to learning and teaching*,[35] Pendleton, Schofield, Tate and Havelock outlined seven tasks in the consultation, and concluded that:

> ... there is no single type or style of relationship which can be identified as more effective than all others. There are, however, certain strategies and skills which can affect both communication in the consultation and sub-sequent outcomes.[35]

They went on to describe such strategies and skills in some detail and to consider learning about and teaching the consultation using consultation tasks (for example, consultation mapping, consultation rating and giving feedback). Although relationships are acknowledged, the focus of the research and teaching is on the strategies and the skills.

Neighbour[36] classified models of the consultation along two axes: doctor centred/patient centred and task orientated/behaviour orientated. In task-orientated models, 'the consultation is viewed as an amalgam of separate and definable tasks, a checklist of points to be covered'. Behaviour-orientated models look 'at the range of behaviours called for within' the consultation. His own 'five checkpoint' model provides points to be visited while journeying through an individual consultation. The focus is on skills to be used in a single interaction. Similarly, in more recent descriptions (for example, the Three Function Approach,[37] the E4 model[38] and the Calgary–Cambridge Guide[39]), the approach is primarily task orientated within individual interactions.

Analysis of the medical consultation (defined as 'the methodic identification, categorisation, and quantification of salient features of doctor–patient communications')[40] also uses observation instruments (or 'interaction analysis systems'). These systems distinguish between *process analysis* and *micro-analysis*.[41] Process analysis involves 'working directly from direct observations or tape recordings of conversations without the use of transcripts'.

Verbal behaviours (such as asking questions, showing approval, voicing affect, giving information) are then sorted and counted. In contrast, microanalytic methods study individual conversations with detailed transcripts of audiotaped or videotaped conversations (for example, discourse analysis,[42] concordancing and conversation analysis[43,44]).

Many models of the consultation, and all the methods of analysis noted, share a common feature in emphasising the doctor–patient encounter as a technical problem of practice which may be understood by analysis and measurement within the individual interaction (looking, for example, at the micro-components of a specific block of time or at specific consultation skills). The strength of these approaches is that they enable analysts, teachers and learners alike to develop behavioural skills that may improve outcomes for both patients and doctors. The weaknesses are first that such models may be given undue priority and become a focus in themselves, blocking attention to wider aspects of professional interactions. Although models may help to 'clarify the basics in communication, (they) never completely capture what happens in reality'.[45] Second, in generally focusing within the individual interaction, some models take little or no account of the longer-term trajectory, or context, of that interaction, the ongoing doctor–patient relationship of which each individual interaction itself forms a micro-component.

In the 1990s, models appeared which aimed to combine both the general nature of early work and specificity or teachability. An example is the six component patient-centred model of Stewart *et al.* (*see* Box below).[45] This model, while emphasising the necessity to attend to cues and use communication skills, builds in a further emphasis on an integrated understanding of the whole person over time (component 2) and on continuity of care in the context of effective long-term relationships with healing potential (component 5). These components point to the longer-term nature, or journey, of many doctor–patient relationships. Similarly, the Kalamazoo Consensus[46] endorses 'a patient-centred or relationship-centred approach ... within and across encounters'.

The six interactive components of the patient-centred process[45]

- Exploring both the disease and the illness experience
  - History, physical, lab
  - Dimensions of illness (ideas, feelings, expectations, effects on function)
- Understanding the whole person
  - The person (for example, life history and personal and developmental issues)

- The proximal context (for example, family, employment, social support)
- The distal context (for example, culture, community, ecosystem)
- Finding common ground
  - Problems and priorities
  - Goals of treatment or management
  - Roles of doctor and patient
- Incorporating prevention and health promotion
  - Health enhancement
  - Risk avoidance
  - Risk reduction
  - Early identification
  - Complication reduction
- Enhancing the doctor–patient relationship
  - Compassion
  - Power
  - Healing
  - Self-awareness
  - Transference and countertransference
- Being realistic
  - Time and timing
  - Wise stewardship of resources
  - Team building and teamwork

The swing from a bedside cosmology of illness to an object-orientated biomedical cosmology[26] in the practice of medicine during the twentieth century has parallels in the study of GP–patient encounters. A swing also occurred from the early writings on GP–patient encounters,[30,32] which focused at a general, relationship level, to later writings[33,35,36,42] that emphasised the technical aspects of the process of communication. I have suggested that the emergence of patient-centredness starts to address the longer-term trajectory and context of the doctor–patient relationship. However, as I describe in the final section which follows, descriptions of patient-centredness are in themselves incomplete, containing inherent limitations and tensions.

Professional ideals and everyday reality

The stories and reflections on my daily work in the Preface may seem obvious or even routine to the reader who is a practising GP, but they hide tensions between the ordinary work of the GP and the ideals of the profession. For example, the *European Definition of General Practice/Family Medicine*[47] gives 11 characteristics of the discipline of general practice, including that it:

- develops a person-centred approach, orientated to the individual, his or her family, and their community
- has a unique consultation process, which establishes a relationship over time, through effective communication between doctor and patient
- is responsible for the provision of longitudinal continuity of care as determined by the needs of the patient
- deals with health problems in their physical, psychological, social, cultural and existential dimensions.

It also adds that GPs will 'utilise the knowledge and trust engendered by repeated contacts'. A report from the Royal College of General Practitioners (RCGP), *The Nature of General Medical Practice*,[48] is clear that the GP needs to practise an art as well as apply medical science, the latter being only one part of patient care. It notes that a consultation should take account not only of disease (the medical model) but also of illness (the social model) and the hopes, fears, feelings and expectations of the patient.

Patients in primary care have been shown to want a patient-centred approach from their GP,[49] a core value[50] advocated in the *European Definition of General Practice/Family Medicine*.[47] Such an approach has been described in the patient-centred clinical method,[45] further developed by Mead and Bower[51] (*see* Box below).

Five conceptual dimensions for patient-centredness[51]

- Biopsychosocial perspective
  - A perspective on illness that includes consideration of social and psychological (as well as biomedical) factors
- 'Patient-as-person'
  - Understanding the personal meaning of the illness for each individual patient
- Sharing power and responsibility
  - Sensitivity to patients' preferences for information and shared decision making, and responding appropriately to these
- Therapeutic alliance
  - Developing common therapeutic goals and enhancing the personal bond between doctor and patient

- The 'doctor-as-person'
  - Awareness of the influence of the personal qualities and subjectivity of the doctor on the practice of medicine

One dimension of patient-centredness is the *therapeutic alliance*,[51] which emerged from Balint's view of the doctor–patient relationship as therapeutic in its own right.[30] This concept, founded on psychotherapeutic notions, is the basis of Balint's well-known aphorism 'the drug doctor'. Balint distinguished between listening in the immediate *interaction* and the ongoing *relationship* built over time:

> The doctor's ... ability to listen to the events as they develop in the doctor patient relationship during the interview ... and the doctor patient relationship in ... its special form as it occurs in general practice and in no other field of medicine. This special form of the doctor patient relationship in general practice is conditioned by the long and intimate connection between the two. We described it as a 'mutual investment company'.[30]

Similarly, for the RCGP, the sick person is thought to expect more than the doctor's scientific training and experience of the ideal GP:

> He will look for something more. He will want the doctor to be interested in him as someone who in the last resort is different from everyone else and not as an example from a herd.[52]

This concept of the 'special' doctor–patient relationship, an alliance which 'has potential therapeutic benefit in and of itself',[51] is integral to both patient-centred medicine and the ideals of general practice.[47] Although there is no doubt that alliances occur in GP–patient interactions, it is less clear how they are applied in pragmatic everyday practice. For example, Balint's assumption of ongoing care by a personal doctor has been questioned in current general practice.[53,54] Some GPs not only see the centre of their work as the diagnosis and treatment of objectifiable organic pathologies,[55] but actively limit involvement in the psychosocial experience of their patients.[56] Similarly, although the importance of agreement over goals of treatment in the doctor–patient relationship has been emphasised,[57] there is little evidence that the related concept of shared decision making actually occurs in routine GP consultations.[58] Tuckett *et al.*[59] concluded that most consultations were one-sided, with limited sharing or exchange of ideas.

Tensions between theoretical and professional ideals and their application in everyday practice are also evident within the patient-centred clinical method[45] itself. An all-encompassing component ('understanding the whole person' – component 2) contrasts with a limiting one ('being realistic' – component 6). The latter involves being realistic in terms of what a single practitioner can reasonably be expected to achieve in providing patient-centred care, including issues of time, team building and the importance of wise stewardship in accessing resources.[45]

Hence GPs must both be available to listen and form a special relationship with each different patient, and at the same time be realistic about what they can reasonably be expected to achieve given their personal human limitations. The tension evident in the literature between professional ideals and the reality of daily work is also apparent in this book.

Conclusion

In this Introduction, I have argued that it is important to utilise and integrate stories or narratives in understanding the everyday world and work of medicine and primary care. I have suggested that the swing from a bedside understanding of illness towards an object-oriented biomedical approach to medical practice has parallels in the study of GP–patient encounters, in which early work focused at a general relational level. Later writings emphasise technical, behavioural and measureable aspects of communication with less focus on the longer-term trajectory and context of GP–patient relationships. I suggest that patient-centredness starts to address these areas but that there remains a significant tension between professional ideals and everyday practice.

This book is based on in-depth accounts from experienced GPs, allowing a picture of doctors' perceptions of their routine everyday work to emerge. In reflecting on these doctors' taken-for-granted world of practice, this book offers insights to GP–patient relationships established over time, the cumulative consequence of numerous individual interactions. The narrative stories of everyday general practice allow exploration of perceptions of choice in listening, of limits and boundaries framing work, and of the doctor's self. A picture emerges of the pragmatic application of patient-centred theory as doctors attempt both to be available (in line with their professional ideals) and to be realistic about availability (as they encounter everyday reality). Although these insights have limitations (as I note in Appendix I), their perspective is both different from, and complementary to, the more behaviour-oriented models and approaches outlined in this Introduction. The material described in this book can in no way be quantified but offers a rich and valid view of primary care and the social and relational context of GP–patient relationships in a semi-rural area of the UK at the start of the twenty-first century.

References

1   Charlton B (1991) Stories of sickness. *Br J Gen Pract.* **41**: 222–3.

2   Montgomery Hunter K (1991) *Doctors' Stories.* Princeton University Press, Princeton.

3   Greenhalgh T, Hurwitz B (1998) *Narrative Based Medicine.* BMJ Books, London.

4   Launer J (2003) Narrative-based medicine: a passing fad or a giant leap for general practice? *Br J Gen Pract.* **53**: 91–2.

5   Jacobson L, Edwards A, Granier S *et al.* (1997) Evidence-based medicine and general practice. *Br J Gen Pract.* **47**: 449–52.

6   Macnaughton J (1995) Anecdotes and empiricism. *Br J Gen Pract.* **45**: 571–2.

7   Brody H (1987) *Stories of Sickness.* Yale University Press, New Haven.

8   Rabin S, Maoz B, Elata-Alster G (1999) Doctors' narratives in Balint groups. *Br J Med Psychol.* **72**: 121–5.

9   Cronin A (1937) *The Citadel.* Victor Gollancz, London.

10 Ferris P (1965) *The Doctors.* Victor Gollancz, London.

11 Berger J, Mohr J (1967) *A Fortunate Man.* Penguin, London.

12 West L (2001) *Doctors on the Edge.* Free Association Books, London.

13 Clark J, Mischler E (1992) Attending to patients' stories: reframing the clinical task. *Soc Health Illness.* **14**: 344–71.

14 Gibson R (1981) *The Family Doctor: his life and history.* George Allen & Unwin, London.

15 Lane K (1982) *Diary of a Medical Nobody.* Corgi, London.

16 Matthews H, Bain J (1998) *Doctors Talking.* Scottish Cultural Press, Edinburgh.

17 Borkan J, Reis S, Steinmetz D, Medalie J (1999) *Patients and Doctors: life-changing stories from primary care.* University of Wisconsin Press, Wisconsin.

18 Borkan J, Miller W, Reis S (1992) Medicine as storytelling. *Fam Pract.* **9**: 127–9.

19 Williams W (1968) *The Autobiography of William Carlos Williams.* MacGibbon & Kee, New York.

20 Williams W (1984) *The Doctor Stories.* New Directions, New York.

21 Goffman E (1969) *The Presentation of Self in Everyday Life.* Penguin, London.

22 Porritt Report (1962) *A Review of the Medical Services in Great Britain.* Social Assay, London.

23 Gillie Report (1963) *The Field of Work of the Family Doctor. Report to the Standing Medical Advisory Committee.* HMSO, London.

24 Hutchison R (1950) Medicine today and yesterday. *BMJ.* **220**: 72–3.

25   Nicholls L (1966) My grandfather's practice. *Lancet.* **2**: 1412–13.

26   Jewson N (1976) The disappearance of the sick-man from medical cosmology. *Sociology.* **10**: 225–44.

27   Fissell M (1991) The disappearance of the patient's narrative and the invention of hospital medicine. In: French R, Wear A (eds) *British Medicine in an Age of Reform.* Routledge, London.

28   May C, Mead N (1999) Patient-centredness: a history. In: Frith L, Dowrick C (eds) *Ethical Issues in General Practice: uncertainty and responsibility.* Routledge, London.

29   Armstrong D (1979). The emancipation of biographical medicine. *Soc Sci Med.* **13A**: 1–8.

30   Balint M (1963) *The Doctor, His Patient and the Illness* (2e). Churchill Livingstone, London.

31   Bower P, Gask L, May C, Mead N (2001) Domains of consultation research in primary care. *Patient Educ Couns.* **45**: 3–11.

32   Browne K, Freeling P (1967) *The Doctor–Patient Relationship.* Livingstone, London.

33   Byrne P, Long B (1976) *Doctors Talking to Patients.* HMSO, London.

34   Byrne P, Heath C (1980) Practitioners' use of non-verbal behaviour in real consultations. *J R Coll Gen Pract.* **30**: 327–31.

35   Pendleton D, Schofield T, Tate P, Havelock P (1984) *The Consultation.* Oxford University Press, Oxford.

36   Neighbour R (1987) *The Inner Consultation.* Petroc Press, Newbury.

37   Cohen-Cole S (1991) *The Medical Interview: the three-function approach.* Mosby, St Louis.

38   Keller V, Carroll J (1994) A new model for physician–patient communication. *Patient Educ Couns.* **23**: 131–40.

39   Silverman J, Kurtz S, Draper J (2005) *Skills for Communicating with Patients* (2e). Radcliffe Publishing, Oxford.

40   Ong L, Haes J, Hoos A, Lammes F (1995) Doctor–patient communication: a review of the literature. *Soc Sci Med.* **40**: 903–18.

41   Charon R, Greene M, Adelman R (1994) Multi-dimensional interaction analysis: a collaborative approach to the study of medical discourse. *Soc Sci Med.* **39**: 995–65.

42   Gwyn R, Elwyn G (1999) When is a shared decision not (quite) a shared decision? Negotiating preferences in a general practice encounter. *Soc Sci Med.* **49**: 437–47.

43   Perakyla A (1997) Conversation analysis: a new model of research in doctor–patient communication. *J R Soc Med.* **90**: 205–8.

44 Skelton J, Wearn A, Hobbs F (2002) 'I' and 'we': a concordancing analysis of how doctors and patients use first person pronouns in primary care consultations. *Fam Pract.* **19**: 484–8.

45 Stewart M, Brown J, Weston W *et al.* (2003) *Patient-centred Medicine* (2e). Radcliffe Medical Press, Oxford.

46 Participants in the Bayer–Fetzer Conference on Physician–Patient Communication in Medical Education (2001) Essential elements of communication in medical encounters: the Kalamazoo Consensus statement. *Acad Med.* **76**: 390–3.

47 WONCA (2002) *The European Definition of General Practice/Family Medicine.* The European Society of General Practice/Family Medicine, Europe.

48 Royal College of General Practitioners (1996) *The Nature of General Medical Practice. Report from General Practice 27.* Royal College of General Practitioners, London.

49 Little P, Everitt H, Williamson I *et al.* (2001) Preferences of patients for patient centred approach to consultation in primary care: observational study. *BMJ.* **322**: 468–72.

50 Howie J, Heaney D, Maxwell M (2004) Quality, core values and the general practice consultation: issues of definition, measurement and delivery. *Fam Pract.* **21**: 458–68.

51 Mead N, Bower P (2000) Patient-centredness: a conceptual framework and review of the empirical literature. *Fam Pract.* **51**: 1087–110.

52 Royal College of General Practitioners (1972) *The Future General Practitioner.* Royal College of General Practitioners, London.

53 Baker R (1997) Will the future GP remain a personal doctor? *Br J Gen Pract.* **47**: 831–4.

54 Hjortdahl P (2001) Continuity of care – going out of style? *Br J Gen Pract.* **51**: 699–700.

55 Dowrick C, May C, Richardson M *et al.* (1996) The biopsychosocial model of general practice: rhetoric or reality? *Br J Gen Pract.* **46**: 105–7.

56 May C, Dowrick C, Richardson M (1996) The confidential patient: the social construction of therapeutic relationships in general medical practice. *Sociological Review.* **44**: 187–203.

57 Roth A, Fonaghy P (1996) *What Works for Whom? A critical review of psychotherapy research.* Guildford, London.

58 Stevenson F, Barry C, Britten N, Barber N, Bradley C (2000) Doctor–patient communication about drugs: the evidence for shared decision making. *Soc Sci Med.* **50**: 829–40.

59 Tuckett D, Boulton M, Olson C, Wiliams A (1985) *Meetings between Experts.* Tavistock, London.

Section 1
Choices in listening

1

The importance of listening

Listening to the patient's story has long been regarded as central to the practice of medicine ('Listen to the patient, he is telling you the diagnosis.').[1] Learning to hear a story is a core skill for any aspiring doctor and more than 85% of diagnoses in medical outpatients may be made from the history and referral letter without further examination or investigation.[2] Listening at the *start* of interactions is integral to models of the consultation (for example, understanding the patient's problem and perspective,[3] connecting,[4] gathering data to understand the patient,[5] engaging the patient and eliciting the story[6]), and forms the basis of much communication teaching, both undergraduate and postgraduate. But listening in medicine is more than simply hearing a story at the start of an interaction, and models also emphasise spotting and responding to patients' cues in order to listen *during* interactions (verbal and non-verbal signals,[7] picking up and checking out cues[8]). In this first Section, I explore GPs' perceptions concerning listening in their everyday work, both initiating listening and choosing *not* to listen during interactions.

The value of listening

The role of the GP as someone who is easily available for talking, offering time and listening within the community is a major theme for these doctors. There is good evidence that this is also valued by patients.[9–11] Listening is important as:

> 'Part of our global approach, social factors, physical factors, psychological factors.' (Matt)

> 'I just let her sit and talk. You've got to set aside time to listen. I think that's part of the importance of being a GP, providing a great big ear sometimes, and nothing more, for patients to talk into. . . . no matter how awkward it is or difficult, I think you've just got to take it on board and sit and listen.' (Steve)

'Her husband suddenly had a massive stroke, so she stopped work to look after him. She finds it very hard and she's very bitter about it. She feels guilty and she off-loaded all this to me and I spent most of the consultation listening. She seemed to feel a bit happier at the end of it, somebody actually taking an interest in it really. I think listening is a big important part of the job. I think we achieve something every time she comes.' (Alex)

'A familiar face that she knows, just to talk about it.' (Ben)

In addition to accessibility, the GP may be the only person to whom patients feel they can turn:

'She just really had nobody else at all to talk to. I had to listen long and I had to listen hard. It all poured out and poured out. I said very little. I see it as within my remit to try and help.' (Chris)

Another, more pragmatic, valuing of listening is that:

'If you don't get to the bottom of why a patient has come to see you, then they just keep coming back.' (Ben)

'It is desperately important to sit there and let them tell the whole story because if you cut them too soon, you will miss vital things. If you actually take the time to listen instead of jumping in and thinking "for heaven's sake, why have they troubled me with this?", you will find out exactly why they are there, because great granny has died or their friend's got this or that.' (Phil)

In other words, listening is essential and 'if you listen for long enough, you will find out the real reason why the patient has attended' (Phil). Another reason for investing time in listening is the long-term effect that it may have on the relationship:

'Patients with demanding multiple trivial complaints. I have had occasions when appropriate listening time has been very relevant for them, probably at some cost to myself. I think those are very draining consultations. Occasionally they've created a very different relationship afterwards. It may just be the opener for many subsequent consultations or it may move the rest of the relationship on to a totally new level.' (Lew)

Time spent listening now is thought to reap rewards in the future and alter the balance of the doctor–patient relationship. Listening is also seen as therapeutic in itself:

'One thing I have realised is how therapeutic listening can be. Just sitting and listening to somebody who comes along with a crisis situation, you might not necessarily think you're the most appropriate person. What you do is you sit and listen for a while and you maybe see them once again afterwards and they're sorting it out. You realise that you've actually done a fair bit of good in quite a short space of time.' (Rick)

There is general agreement that listening is appropriate, important and a good use of time:

'Giving space and listening is what makes me a GP.' (Sam)

'We are there to listen.' (Tim)

The idealising tone of these responses contrasts with the similar consensus that spending time listening can be hard and frustrating, and may produce problems:

'It's much easier to give a prescription than it is to actually listen to people.' (Pete)

'We don't always have the answers.' (Ed)

'I would say 50% of consultations need some exploration away from the purely physical. . . . as important as handing them a prescription. The problem is, it's very time-consuming but it's quite satisfying so I do quite a lot of it.' (Sam)

Finding the time for listening and the limits these doctors establish will be explored later in this section.

When discussing listening, the themes explored were not around specific skills but about aspects of relationship and knowing patients in a wider sense:

'I think good listening skills are about risking something in a relationship to become more involved.' (Lew)

'Where I come from people regard their doctor as, not threatening, but somebody on a completely different level to you, and I think maybe find it hard to go to the doctor and actually communicate effectively with them – in awe of them. So I thought "If you're trying to be a good doctor, you've got to try and be approachable and reassuring to people that what they're telling you isn't ridiculous, and they can feel able to just tell you whatever they want".' (Vic)

'So I just sat back and let it all come at me for a while and let her get it off her chest. I was quite pleased that she could feel that kind of anger.' (Rick)

'In general practice you interact really, you live in the locality, work in the locality and I think just getting the listening skills – the verbal clues – ask another question ... ask "what's going on at home, what's going on with your children, what's going on at work?" and be prepared, once you've asked that question, just to sit back in your chair and listen.' (Matt)

Recognising that listening is needed

For these GPs, recognising that someone needs listening and attention, in the form of time to talk during the consultation in the middle of a busy surgery, is part of day-to-day life and work. How this recognition of need actually occurs varies from doctor to doctor, from patient to patient and from context to context. Sometimes the doctor may simply 'realise' that listening is needed:

'You'll start off, someone will come in with something quite straightfor-ward and all of a sudden will say something and you'll realise that that's not really the problem. That's a starter for ten sort of thing and then if they're feeling confident with you and relaxed and maybe you've demonstrated some listening skills, they will then tell you what the real problem is.' (Vic)

Recognition may be a natural consequence of a consultation about a physical problem:

'A lady came in really requesting a repeat prescription for omeprazole and to ask about gastroscopy. She then got on to her holiday and that in turn led to how she'd met someone, which in turn led to her ongoing problems with bereavement. She lost her son a long time ago.' (Pat)

From Pat's account, it seems that there was a progression from present and physical issues to longstanding and underlying issues. The common ground and ongoing relationship already established in previous consultations, and the safety of having started with a physical issue, appear to have given space and confidence within the consultation for a longstanding and deep problem to be aired. In contrast, the situation is seen as different with a patient not previously known to the GP:

'If you have a brand new patient with a brand new problem, then I think you've got to be open and, particularly if you haven't got a clue what's going on, you've got to try and let it come.' (Huw)

Without the common ground of previous relationship, extra vigilance is required to hear all the different aspects of the story. In the long term, that patience and attention to full listening reap rewards in terms of trust and sharing – the relationship starts to become established.

The listening GP must first of all, and as an essential prerequisite for listening, spot the cues given by the patient that listening is needed, and be alert to the possibility that:

'It's the hidden agenda – they are coming in with something, but while they are there ...' (Phil)

Similarly, some people:

'Have physical problems and they use the physical problem as a currency to deal with the general practitioner.' (Ed)

The difficulty is differentiating the purely physical problem from the physical problem being used as a ticket to consult about other issues.

Spotting cues as the consultation proceeds has long been recognised in the literature of general practice as part of the doctor's work (for example, Balint[12]), as part of the 'physician's clinical instinct'.[13] Levinson et al. define a cue as 'a direct or indirect comment that provides information about any aspect of a patient's life circumstances or feelings'.[14] Cues come in a variety of guises and can point to a variety of issues for the patient (not just a physical illness). They can be verbal or non-verbal[15] and are easy to miss (sometimes with devastating consequences[16]). They can occur at any stage in the consultation and require skill to perceive what is hinted at, missed out or skirted round. Tonge[17] has called this 'listening with the third ear', which resonates with Neighbour's[4] analogy of the doctor having two heads. Cues may be quite overt (but easily ignored):

'Somebody comes in with some symptoms and you perhaps are just contemplating this and they all of a sudden come out with "Could this for example be stress-related, doctor?" And the next question is "Well why do you ask a question like that?".' (Will)

The person who makes an aside during[18] or just as they are leaving the consultation ('the dreaded doorway question'[19]) is also well recognised in general practice:[20,21]

'I sometimes note the hand on the door handle as they go out – the aside – and you have to drag them back. That's what they've really come for. Sometimes they're conscious of what they've really come for, sometimes they're not.' (Don)

Cues do not have to be spoken out loud:

'I suppose really she came with two specific symptoms but behind it, there was a whole host of other things. It was just her body language as well. Her body language suggested to me that it wasn't just that she was forgetting things. Her pressure of speech was there and she was sitting on the edge of her seat and a bit agitated. She wasn't relaxed.' (Vic)

Cues noted by these doctors are summarised in Box 1.1. They include how people present themselves in the consultation, and all aspects of their body language, dress, manner and demeanour.

Box 1.1 Doctors' examples of patients' cues indicating that listening is needed

- Body language and dress (for example, sitting on the edge of the seat, general appearance)
- Manner and demeanour (for example, pressure of speech, agitation)
- Frequency of attendance (for example, 'somebody who comes once a year suddenly appears three times in a fortnight with something trivial')
- The patient who asks, 'Could this be stress-related, doctor?'
- The person who makes an aside just as they are leaving the consultation
- The person who does not want to give detail about certain symptoms
- The patient who demands attention, 'I think my husband's got cancer'

Other cues may not be quite so obvious:

'You know something is not right just by the way that somebody who comes once a year suddenly appears three times in a fortnight with something trivial. You know that it's not them and I think I can say to them "Look, what's going on? Usually you come once a year, suddenly you're here and it doesn't seem that important. What's underlying this?".' (Don)

'A lady came and said she wasn't feeling terribly well, was feeling a bit down, yet didn't appear to want to go into it in any more detail. So you get this sort of hunch at times. It began to come out that her husband had left her ...' (Steve)

The cue may be in what is left unsaid[18] or it may be the patient who recognises that listening is needed, which demands attention in the consultation:

'She talked about two minor problems before, "Oh, by the way, I think I should mention, I think my husband's got cancer".' (Lew)

'We talked about her arm. "I think I'm pregnant" were her next words. And she was 16, broken family, unable to talk to her mum. Hadn't had a period for two months and as she was talking about her past and current problems, her level of anxiety just seemed to lift and dissipate.' (Adam)

Cues are well recognised in the literature[8] and Lang *et al.*[22] have described a useful taxonomy.

- Expression of feelings (especially concern, fear or worry) – verbal or non-verbal.
- Attempts to explain or understand symptoms.
- Speech clues that underscore particular concerns of the patient (for example, repetition or pauses).
- Sharing a personal story that links the patient with medical conditions or risks.
- Behaviour clues suggesting unresolved concerns or expectations (for example, reluctance to accept recommendations, seeking a second opinion, early return visit).

Apart from spotting cues as a consultation proceeds, the simplest way of recognising that listening is needed is allowing the patient uninterrupted space to talk at the start of the interaction:

'I try and sit back in my chair, rather than leaning forward, or turn the chair to face the patient, and adopt an open posture rather than a closed one. Sometimes I move a little closer. I try really hard to put my hands on the chair and sit back and not keep interrupting them and not keep firing questions at them. To actually let them get through what they want to get through rather than doing a normal history where you are forever asking questions and expecting answers.' (Jo)

'We have a policy, apart from the opening gambit of "How are you?" or "Hello", or whatever, at the beginning of every consultation to actually keep our mouth shut for at least 30 seconds, at least.' (Alex)

Although this sounds simple, translating 'knowing' into 'doing'[23] or 'technical-rational knowledge' into 'knowing-in-action'[24] is difficult in everyday work. Despite the theoretical emphasis on spotting cues noted earlier, studies of doctor–patient interactions are clear that patients' cues are frequently missed or not acknowledged by doctors,[14,25–27] even though this may result in longer consultations.[14] Beckman and Frankel[28] showed that patients were interrupted by their physicians in primary care so soon after describing their presenting problems (on average within 18 seconds) that they failed to disclose other significant concerns. In contrast, Blau[29] deliberately let patients in a neuro-logical clinic speak uninterrupted, at the start of the consultation, until 'the end of the account was indicated by a cessation of speech, a look on the patient's face, or a concluding statement'. Seventy per cent of patients spoke for two minutes or less, and the overall average was less than two minutes. These results are supported by a similar study of spontaneous talking time at the start of the consultation from the outpatient clinic of a Swiss tertiary referral centre[30] (mean spontaneous talking time was 92 seconds, 78% of patients had finished their initial statement in two minutes). A similar study in pri-mary care[31] showed a mean initial monologue length, when uninterrupted, of 28 seconds. It would seem that allowing space at the start of the consultation may not take an inordinate amount of time. Alex's comment above is typical of several of these doctors who attempt to give their patients such adequate time at the start of the consultation, noting that, unless they do, they 'don't get to the bottom' (Ben) of their patient's agenda:

Identification of the patient's agenda lies at the very heart of the consultation. It is not an optional extra.[32]

Unvoiced agenda items lead to poor outcomes,[33] but actively eliciting patients' concerns improves patient satisfaction.[34] As most patients come to the consultation with a particular agenda[32] and with more than one concern to discuss,[35–38] failure to address this agenda and these concerns is likely to adversely affect the outcome of this interaction and also subsequent health-care outcomes.

Recognising when listening is needed to hear someone's agenda is central to listening work. Both conscious acknowledgement of listening as important work and conscious competence in identifying cues or making space are implicit in this work. But spotting the hunch, the verbal cue or the body language is seen as only the first step:

'Sometimes, the clues are there and you either choose to pick up on the clues or ignore the clues or sometimes you defer them.' (Huw)

A judgement has to be made (to 'pick up or ignore'), which I explore in the next two chapters.

References

1 Osler W (1904) The master-word in medicine. In: *Aequanimitas, with Other Addresses to Medical Students, Nurses, and Practitioners of Medicine.* Blakiston, Philadelphia.

2 Hampton JR, Harrison MJG, Mitchell JRA *et al.* (1975) Relative contributions of history taking, physical examination and laboratory investigation to diagnosis and management of medical outpatients. *BMJ.* **271**: 486–9.

3 Pendleton D, Schofield T, Tate P *et al.* (2003) *The New Consultation.* Oxford University Press, Oxford.

4 Neighbour R (2004) *The Inner Consultation* (2e). Radcliffe Publishing, Oxford.

5 Cohen-Cole S (1991) *The Medical Interview: the three-function approach.* Mosby, St Louis.

6 Keller V, Carroll J (1994) A new model for physician–patient communication. *Patient Educ Couns.* **23**: 131–40.

7 Stewart M, Brown J, Weston W *et al.* (2003) *Patient-centred Medicine* (2e). Radcliffe Medical Press, Oxford.

8 Silverman J, Kurtz S, Draper J (2005) *Skills for Communicating with Patients* (2e). Radcliffe Publishing, Oxford.

9 Ware J, Snyder M, Wright R (1984) Defining and measuring patient satisfaction with medical care. *Eval Prog Plan.* **6**: 247–63.

10 Williams S, Calnan M (1991) Key determinants of consumer satisfaction with general practice. *Fam Pract.* **8**: 237–42.

11 Wensing M, Jung H, Mainz J *et al.* (1998) A systematic review of the literature on patient priorities for general practice care. Part 1: description of the research domain. *Soc Sci Med.* **47**: 1573–88.

12 Balint M (1963) *The Doctor, His Patient and the Illness* (2e). Churchill Livingstone, London.

13 Mackenzie J, cited in Abercrombie G (1959) The art of the consultation. *J Coll Gen Pract.* **2**: 15–21.

14 Levinson W, Gorawara-Bhat R, Lamb J (2000) A study of patient clues and physician responses in primary care and surgical settings. *JAMA.* **284**: 1021–7.

15   Byrne P, Heath C (1980) Practitioners' use of non-verbal behaviour in real consultations. *J R Coll Gen Pract.* **30**: 327–31.

16   Last J (2000) Distress symptoms may be easy to miss. *BMJ.* **320**: 717.

17   Tonge W (1967) Listening with the third ear. *J Coll Gen Pract.* **62**(suppl 3): 13–17.

18   Matthews D, Suchman A, Branch W (1993) Making connexions: enhancing the therapeutic potential of patient–clinician relationships. *Ann Intern Med.* **118**: 973–7.

19   Roter D, Hall J (1992) *Doctors Talking with Patients/Patients Talking with Doctors.* Auburn House, Westport.

20   Browne K, Freeling P (1967) *The Doctor–Patient Relationship.* Livingstone, London.

21   White J, Levinson W, Roter D (1994) 'Oh by the way ...': the closing moments of the medical visit. *J Gen Intern Med.* **9**: 24–8.

22   Lang F, Floyd M, Beine K (2000) Clues to patients' explanations and concerns about their illnesses. *Arch Fam Med.* **9**: 222–7.

23   Miller G (1990) The assessment of clinical skills/competence/performance. *Acad Med (suppl).* **65**: S63–S70.

24   Schon D (1983) *The Reflective Practitioner.* Temple Smith, London.

25   Tuckett D, Boulton M, Olson C *et al.* (1985) *Meetings between Experts: an approach to sharing ideas in medical consultations.* Tavistock, London.

26   Suchman A, Markakis K, Beckman H *et al.* (1997) A model of empathic communication in the medical interview. *JAMA.* **277**: 678–82.

27   Campion P, Foulkes J, Neighbour R *et al.* (2002) Patient centredness in the MRCGP video examination: analysis of large cohort. *BMJ.* **325**: 691–2.

28   Beckman H, Frankel R (1984) The effect of physician behaviour on the collection of data. *Ann Intern Med.* **101**: 692–6.

29   Blau J (1989) Time to let the patient speak. *BMJ.* **298**: 39.

30   Langewitz W, Denz M, Keller A *et al.* (2002) Spontaneous talking time at start of consultation in outpatient clinic: cohort study. *BMJ.* **325**: 682–3.

31   Rabinowitz I, Luzzati R, Tamir A *et al.* (2004) Length of patient's monologue, rate of completion, and relation to other components of the clinical encounter: observational intervention study in primary care. *BMJ.* **328**: 501–2.

32   McKinley R, Middleton J (1999) What do patients want from doctors? Content analysis of written patient agendas for the consultation. *Br J Gen Pract.* **49**: 796–800.

33   Barry C, Bradley CP, Britten N *et al.* (2000) Patients' unvoiced agendas in general practice consultations: qualitative study. *BMJ.* **320**: 1246–50.

34 Maclean M, Armstrong D (2004) Eliciting patients' concerns: an RCT of different approaches by the doctor. *Br J Gen Pract.* **54**: 663–6.

35 Starfield B, Wray C, Hess K *et al.* (1981) The influence of patient practitioner agreement on outcome of care. *Am J Pub Health.* **71**: 127–31.

36 Good M, Good B (1982) *Patient Requests in Primary Care Clinics.* D Reidel, Boston.

37 Wasserman R, Inui T, Barriatua R *et al.* (1984) Pediatric clinicians' support for parents makes a difference. *Pediatrics.* **6**: 1047–53.

38 Greenfield S, Kaplan S, Ware J (1985) Expanding patient involvement in care. *Ann Intern Med.* **102**: 520–8.

2

Choosing to listen

Once it is identified that listening is needed, a choice has to be made (to 'pick up or ignore') which is central to the listening work of the GP:

'Sometimes, the clues are there and you either choose to pick up on the clues or ignore the clues or sometimes you defer them.' (Huw)

'If somebody comes in and says "I've got a pain in my chest" and then it comes out that they are really worrying about their wife's dementia or something. … You've perhaps been rattling along, aware that you are running late or whatever, and you're sticking to, I was going to say protocols but that's not the right word, but tramlines. When somebody comes in with chest pain, there are two or three questions you always ask about it, "Where is it? When does it happen? Have you tried anything for it?" and you've not really sat there and listened to them telling you in their own words and when they drop something into what they are saying and you suddenly think "Oh goodness me, I'm rushing the patient, I'd better stop … .". So I usually put the pen down, uncross my legs and say "Just tell me in your own words about it" or whatever. Like an apology that I'm rushing them perhaps.' (Tim)

Being stuck in the tramlines of almost routine 'chest pain questions' contrasts with the choice of whether or not to loop down an alternative route and spend time listening:

'The person who comes in with a presenting complaint. Then you get the verbal or visual clue that there's something else going on and you make a decision as to whether you're able to go on that loop. You think how late you are running and what kind of established relationship you may have with that patient already. You take those factors quickly into account and decide whether you're happy to set off down the loop. It seems a bit hard to say that you might actually not set off down the loop, when it's manifestly where they need to be going.' (Rick)

Going into the loop is clearly described:

> 'When you gather that they need to talk, you adopt the posture and body language to allow them to talk. I try and switch into my psychiatry mode to literally encourage them to talk and bring out what they want to do.' (Pete)

Carl May and I have called this tramline metaphor of listening or not listening in doctor–patient interactions the 'listening loop'.[1] It is demonstrated diagrammatically in Figure 2.1, and may be defined as 'a definite period of listening by the GP within the interaction, generally separate to hearing the patient's initial story'. In other words, the loop is a patch of active listening,

Not identifying the points – no cues are spotted so the possibility of a listening loop does not arise:

Identifying the points by spotting cues but choosing not to take a listening loop:

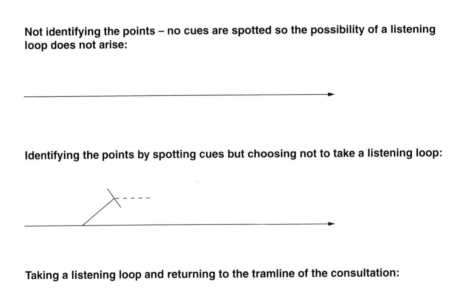

Taking a listening loop and returning to the tramline of the consultation:

Taking a listening loop and finishing the consultation at a different destination:

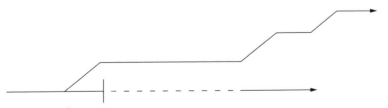

Figure 2.1   The listening loop.

in response to a cue, in addition to the listening required at the start of a consultation to hear the patient's presenting complaint.

The usefulness of the listening loop may be in defining that moment when an interaction might divert from the 'tramline' of a 'biomedical' consultation and take an alternative route. Such moments have been described as 'branch points'[2] or 'windows of opportunity',[3] and judgements concerning them (whether or not to divert or loop) have been being made for years in primary care and elsewhere. The listening loop focuses on this judgement and on factors which emerge from its analysis, particularly resistance to listening by doctors, which I discuss in the next chapter.

Almost all these doctors feel that such loops occur regularly in their work. Also noted is the possibility of more than one loop in an interaction. The few doctors not identifying listening loops feel they listen at the start of the consultation, while hearing the story. After that, they generally ask direct questions and control the interaction:

> 'I think probably in my consultations, the listening tends to be at the beginning. Rightly or wrongly, I tend to sort of consciously try and not direct the consultation and sit back and see what flows initially and then, when I've got a better idea, I'll then start to ask more direct questions. I suppose sometimes the risk you run there is that you haven't got it all before you start jumping in and asking your direct questions. Occasionally there will be another patch where you suddenly realise "Look there's something else here" and then you sit back again. But I must admit that the average consultation is probably a period of listening at the beginning and then me filling in the gaps to enable me to come to some sort of understanding of what's going on.' (Paul)

The tramline metaphor of listening or not listening during a doctor–patient interaction involves:

- *Identifying* the points – spotting a cue which raises the possibility of leaving the initial route or tramline of the consultation.
- *Choosing* to change the points – resulting in an alternative route. Equally importantly, a judgement may be made *not* to change the points.
- *Journeying* down the listening loop route – may involve 'stops'.
- *Ending* the consultation, or journey – may entail return to the initial tramline of the interaction or an alternative destination.

Considerations emerging from the metaphor include the observation that a journey using an alternative route may be longer, shorter or more varied than the original route. Second, stopping places along the way are different and the destination may change (at the anticipated station or elsewhere). Third, the consultation is seen as a journey, a metaphor explored by Neighbour.[4] Lastly, it is difficult to compare the quality of different routes: the most apparently direct may be quicker but will not cover the same ground, and the route which initially seemed best may turn out to be less important than the alternative.

Naming and defining the listening loop (Box 2.1) allows a simple picture of a complex process, 'a taxing part of professional judgement (which) should not occur by default'.[5]

Box 2.1   The listening loop

Definition:
A definite period of listening by the GP within the interaction, generally separate to hearing the patient's initial story.

The loop involves:
- an attitude of being prepared to listen
- spotting cues that such listening may be needed
- a judgement whether or not to set off into the listening
- using listening skills to initiate, sustain and end this patch of listening

---

Prerequisites for diverting and using a listening loop are recognition and listening skills, attitude and choice. First, the ability to recognise or spot cues and generate a conscious awareness that listening may be needed for this patient. Following this recognition, a choice is required which may be made under pressure in the constrained time of the everyday interaction, influenced by a variety of factors − I discuss these in the next chapter. Listening skills for beginning, sustaining and ending interactions are needed.[6−9] The loop adds to these listening skills (common to both counselling and medical interactions) a focus on judgement concerning the explicit initiation of a listening segment within an interaction. The choice of whether or not to listen and take a loop can only take place if the doctor has an attitude of being prepared to spend time and to listen. By implication, this attitude values time spent listening and attending to the 'whole' person in a broad approach to each patient's primary healthcare. Although it may be difficult to teach, such an attitude emerges as central to these doctors' perceptions of their work. Nevertheless, recognising or spotting cues is central − only then can listening and further exploration occur. As already noted, there is evidence that cues are often missed or not acknowledged by doctors in primary care and elsewhere,[2,10–12] suggesting a learning need. The listening loop may help increase skills for conscious awareness of cues.

Choosing to listen during an interaction is important for patients. Just 17% of psychosocial problems in one study[13] were reported in the opening segment of the consultation (a worrying statistic for those doctors who report only offering space for listening at the start of the consultation). The majority of the disclosures occurred after the opening segment, 'when physicians were engaged in taking histories, performing physicals or discussing treatment recommendations for somatic problems',[13] and were facilitated by the doctor specifically enquiring. It should be noted that patients welcome such enquiries.[14] Maintaining attention after the opening phase of the consultation and being prepared to use a listening loop might take listening further and enable discussion of the remaining 83% of psychosocial issues.[13]

In this chapter, I have described the listening loop, a model of choice in listening. It is not a model *of* the consultation but offers an essentially practical description of a common process of choice *within* the interaction that occurs regularly in everyday general practice work after a cue from a patient has been picked up or spotted. In the listening loop, the crucial moment is the judgement, made under pressure in the constrained time of the everyday interaction, of whether or not to start listening in response to the cue by changing the points and taking the loop. Although it has emerged from primary care, it seems likely that a focus on judgements in listening (or not listening) will also be useful in other listening settings. No single model can fully convey the complexity of the doctor–patient encounter,[15] but in most models there is generally an underlying assumption or ideal that listening work is necessary and always occurs when needed. This is not the case in the everyday work of these doctors as I explore in the next chapter – being prepared to use a listening loop brings into view the possibility of *not* using the loop, of limiting listening.

References

1   Cocksedge S, May C (2005) The listening loop: a model of choice about cues within primary care consultations. *Medical Education*. In press.

2   Levinson W, Gorawara-Bhat R, Lamb J (2000) A study of patient clues and physician responses in primary care and surgical settings. *JAMA*. **284**: 1021–7.

3   Branch W, Malik T (1993) Using 'windows of opportunities' in brief interviews to understand patients' concerns. *JAMA*. **269**: 1667–8.

4   Neighbour R (2004) *The Inner Consultation* (2e). Radcliffe Publishing, Oxford.

5   Stewart M, Brown J, Weston W *et al.* (2003) *Patient-centred Medicine* (2e). Radcliffe Medical Press, Oxford.

6   Egan G (1975) *The Skilled Helper.* Brooks/Cole, Monterey.

7   Culley S (1991) *Integrative Counselling Skills in Action.* Sage, London.

8   Feltham C, Horton I (2000) *Handbook of Counselling and Psychotherapy.* Sage, London.

9   Silverman J, Kurtz S, Draper J (2005) *Skills for Communicating with Patients* (2e). Radcliffe Publishing, Oxford.

10 Tuckett D, Boulton M, Olson C *et al.* (1985) *Meetings between Experts: an approach to sharing ideas in medical consultations.* Tavistock, London.

11 Suchman A, Markakis K, Beckman H *et al.* (1997) A model of empathic communication in the medical interview. *JAMA.* **277**: 678–82.

12 Campion P, Foulkes J, Neighbour R *et al.* (2002) Patient centredness in the MRCGP video examination: analysis of large cohort. *BMJ.* **325**: 691–2.

13 Robinson J, Roter D (1999) Psychosocial problem disclosure by primary care patients. *Soc Sci Med.* **48**: 1353–62.

14 Cape J, McCulloch Y (1999) Patients' reasons for not presenting emotional problems in general practice consultations. *Br J Gen Pract.* **49**: 875–9.

15 Freeling P, Gask L (1998) Sticks and stones. *BMJ.* **317**: 1028–9.

3

Choosing not to listen

So far in this section, I have discussed the importance of listening, conscious competence in recognising cues and the listening loop. Although the intrinsic value put on listening in everyday primary care is evident, situations have also been noted in which doctors choose not to listen and put boundaries on their willingness to spend time listening. In this chapter, I consider the pragmatic choices and limits on listening that are employed in the pressure of everyday practice.

Limits on listening: time pressure

Judgements about 'sorting it now', 'getting them to come back' or 'I can't do that today' are part of everyday work for these doctors. The pressures of making the time to listen are acknowledged almost in the same breath as recognition that listening and listening loops occur regularly in day-to-day general practice. These include pressures within the practice to stick to appointment times, trying to find time to listen in emergency consultations, coping with patients who bring lists of problems, and pressures within the doctor such as tiredness or low mood ('having a bad day'), external pressures (such as from the doctor's family – discussed further in Chapter 10), feeling bored or unfulfilled by listening, or guilt at the inability to listen fully. By far the most common reason for choosing not to listen is the pressure of lack of time:

> 'It can be quite hard when you are in a busy surgery and you know that really you need to listen, to sit back and not direct things, but at the same time you can't help but have one eye on the clock and think "I am running late, there are going to be patients out there getting a bit irritated". Sometimes, perhaps for that very reason, you sort of try and tie things up earlier than you would have done under ideal circumstances. But that is just part of the job really, you have to try and judge when you can afford to do that and when it is not a good idea to do it.' (Paul)

'Little consultations can become big ones very, very easily.' (Ben)

'You just let them expand, a river or a tree, it can branch out in any direction, and suddenly you find yourself with this forest. ... Time imposes the pressure and dictates how we consult.' (Huw)

'Listening consultations tend to be long.' (Alex)

A major pressure constantly in the doctor's mind during any consultation is the feeling that people are having to wait for a long time in the waiting room:

'She came in, about the third patient, and spent 40 minutes with me. So you can see the pressure I had with people waiting, and the pressure was building.' (Chaz)

This affects the ability to listen:

'When you are running late, it is very difficult to listen. You still do it, but perhaps not with quite the intensity as early on in the surgery.' (Jo)

There are many situations where listening does not occur, the conscious decision being taken to put the listening to one side. There are also situations where the listening is just left:

'There are times when I don't listen but, usually, I am aware that I am not and there is a reason behind it. It is either because I really think it is not going to be relevant or I'm running late. There must be many other occasions when I am not aware of it.' (Chris)

Other limits on listening

Although pressure of time is very significant, a variety of other factors also influence the judgement to limit listening or categorise listening as inappropriate (*see* Box 3.1). For example, the context in which the listening may or may not take place:

'He stops me at the bottom of the garden and in the street. Maybe that's why I curtailed the conversation.' (Phil)

'It's a bad time, we are two doctors down, so problems that normally we'd spend time for are simply shelved. I can't think of anyone recently where I have deliberately given space to expand.' (Tom)

Box 3.1 Examples of factors that limit listening

- Perceived lack of time
- Work pressures (for example, colleagues absent)
- Doctor's mood
- Doctor's feelings about the patient (for example, likeability or gender)
- Context (for example, emergency surgery appointment, in the street or the garden)
- Patients with apparently insoluble problems
- Patients who may form inappropriate attachments to doctors

Similarly, cancer-phobia was explored with a patient, apparently successfully, in a difficult context:

> 'Just by giving her space, a 12-minute consultation, her anxieties and fears were opened up in terms of her cancer-phobia and all the rest of it. A little bit of space and she's gone, hopefully reassured. It was a totally inappropriate use of time in an emergency appointment.' (Tom)

Appropriate listening space was created in the inappropriate context of a brief emergency appointment.

Factors in the doctor and the patient, such as likeability and gender, also influence the interaction:

> 'The switching off depends on what sort of a day I've had and what type of patient comes in and to a certain extent, whether I find the patient likeable.' (Lee)

> 'A male patient came in to see me whose first words were "I didn't know they made doctors like you," and immediately the barriers went up and I felt very, very uncomfortable.' (Lee)

In response to her patient, this female doctor limited her listening from the first seconds of the consultation.

Another issue is the mood of the GP at the time. Many of these doctors acknowledge that they get tired, grumpy, stretched, busy and pressurised. What sort of mood they are in will affect how they are with their patients that day:

'If I'm very relaxed and happy, I'm probably having a very good surgery, sorting out all the problems in the world. Other days, it's "Are there any useful investigations to do to hold this problem for a couple of weeks?".' (Will)

In some patients, problems are seen to be largely insoluble:

'It was an unsatisfactory consultation but how could I improve it? I just can't imagine myself ever devoting enough time to sort out problems there. I would have to have several consultations of over an hour, and I still don't think we would get anywhere with these issues. She is a chronically anxious soul and lots of people have tried to listen to her, I suspect.' (Adam)

Other patients present slightly different difficulties:

'There are other people who come in and you wouldn't want to just sit back and let them talk all the time because they'd come back and do it every week and you wouldn't make any progress at all and you have to decide what's fair on you and the other people out in the waiting room.' (Rick)

A few doctors raised concerns that attachments might form between patients and their doctors:

'I'll perhaps give them one or two listening consultations but I'm not prepared to take them on for longer because I think they can get glued to you.' (Sam)

'I think the threat in that situation would be if I felt there were some sort of emotional attachment building to me in an inappropriate way.' (Tom)

These fears clearly represent boundaries laid down by a few individual doctors and were not expressed by the majority of those interviewed. I consider the issue of dependency more fully in Chapter 7.

As we have seen, limits on listening vary according to context and situation. However, there is unanimous agreement that in terminal care, all boundaries and limits on listening and time are revised and generally disappear:

'Very definitely, I don't think that I've got limits in the bereavement situation or the planned terminal care situation or, if I have, I haven't found them.' (Tom)

'It is one of the bits in the job where you can actually go the extra mile – perhaps go in the evening or when you're not at work – because you've just got one chance.' (Jo)

Methods of limiting listening

Methods of limiting, blocking or resisting listening work are summarised in Box 3.2. They include allowing the mind to wander, changing the subject, making a plan and using a 'brick wall':

'I obviously wasn't listening, but I gave the time, nodded appropriately, and let my mind wander while he just went on. So I gave the impression of listening, but I wasn't listening because I can't recall it now.' (Adam)

'I would find a pause in the conversation and change the subject to try and shut somebody up. It's something you do without thinking. Interrupt them, politely if possible, or body language. We've got patients who never stop talking and you have to be quite forthright with them. There are occasions when I've actually stood up and said "Thank you for coming, we'll see you next week". I do tend to cut them short.' (Alex)

'Interrupting them, saying "Right, let's do this" and saying something concrete and specific and then they realise that's the end and off they go.' (Steve)

'There are times when I consciously block. You can either do it in an honest, overt way, and say "There just isn't time to get into this at the moment, would you mind coming back with that problem?". Which I am not very good at doing. Or, if you are fairly certain that it has no significance and it is safe to just somehow brush it away, by making a reassuring remark, "I wouldn't worry about that, I'm sure that's fine". Something like that closes it down.' (Chris)

'I tend to start using a brick wall. Very definite disincentives to them wanting to come back. My body language and what I'm telling them all start to be a little less sympathetic and I say "I don't think there is anything more I can actually help you with". It becomes a fairly directed event.' (Tom)

Box 3.2   Methods of limiting, blocking or resisting listening work

- Deferring listening to another time, with the agreement of the patient
- Reassuring
- Changing the subject
- Interrupting
- Nodding appropriately but allowing the mind to wander
- Using body language (such as standing up, a closed posture)
- Reducing sympathy
- Being directive
- Making a plan

These techniques, active and passive, are ways of controlling the workload of listening. Similar strategies, in response to emotional cues from patients in cancer care, have been described as 'blocking behaviours'[1] (*see* Box 3.3).

Box 3.3   Blocking behaviours[1]

- Offering advice and reassurance before the main problems have been identified
- Explaining away distress as normal
- Attending to physical aspects only
- Switching the topic
- 'Jollying' patients along

Sharing listening

Knowing when to share listening with another member of the primary care team is felt to be one of the skills required of the GP:

'If it is purely non-physical, I try to get them off to counselling services. Having discovered that there is a problem then I do try and refer them on if I can't sort it in a couple of sessions and they aren't a physical problem. I refer them on because I just find I'll sink otherwise. I think we do need counselling services and they're probably better at it than me and they have the time.' (Sam)

These doctors use other people to help with listening if they themselves are unable to help patients in a reasonable period of time. This is seen as sometimes a relief for the GP and as a positive benefit for the patient. Although the majority of patients are thought to be happy to be referred, some (often older patients) do not wish to see the counsellor or another member of the primary care team. Similarly, there is a group of patients who see the counsellor once and come back to the GP saying 'That's not for me doctor.' These GPs do not feel particularly skilled in this direction, but accept that this is going to happen and are mostly happy to support their patients in these situations:

'I give a big sigh when I realise that I'm going to be the counsellor.' (Chaz)

'I do the best I can.' (Pete)

'They need a counsellor with medical training.' (Chaz)

'You can't discard them. I always say to them "You can come and see me if it doesn't work, and as often as you want".' (Vic)

'I think it's reasonable that they should come back and see me. I don't remember it causing me a problem. It means they get a different approach. They don't get an in-depth counselling approach, but they do get a chat about their problems and hopefully some sort of support through whatever is bothering them.' (Ben)

The main concern is that doctors do not see themselves as the best people to help in these situations. They all worry about their lack of skills, but some are happy to 'just keep plugging away' (Chaz) if this gives the patient freedom of choice, and 'someone who they gel with, personality-wise' (Phil). Others do not wish to be seen as a 'counselling substitute' or to take patients on for more than one or two consultations. What happens to the patients affected by these various management options is unclear:

'I think the people who don't want to go to the counsellor fall into two groups. There are the ones who are then willing to continue seeing me, and talk to me almost in place of the counsellor, and the ones who don't want to talk much at all, who really just don't want to open up. ... I go on seeing them and what tends to happen is they either stop coming, get better or adjust in some way. Some of them start to open up a bit with me or come round to the idea of seeing the counsellor. But you do get a definite group who say "Oh no, I couldn't do that sort of thing, talking about it would just make it worse". Then you try and get across to them that maybe it might be a bit upsetting at the time but maybe it will make them feel better. It is in those situations that I sometimes feel a bit uneasy because I just wonder "Am I really right? Am I going to make it worse for them?". Obviously there are some people where if you start talking about things, it upsets them a lot more and they don't always come out of it that well. And that's maybe where I'm lacking the counsellor's touch.' (Paul)

If patients are reluctant to see the counsellor, these doctors perceive that it is their role to step in and provide ongoing support, even when they feel there are limits to their skills. There is an unspoken assumption that it is always the GP who is there to pick up the pieces.

Patients and not listening

As this book is based on doctors' accounts, it is hard fully to assess the patient's influence on decision making about listening. However, some clues are available. When results of analyses of patient satisfaction literature are put together (*see* Box 3.4), the common themes (which have been the foundation of much succeeding research) are immediately apparent. The perspective of patients is that their relationship with the doctor ranks alongside the doctor's technical or professional competence in delivery of care when assessing their priorities for, and satisfaction with, their healthcare (although whether patients can truly separate the quality of technical and interpersonal care is debated).[2,3]

Box 3.4 Themes in the patient satisfaction literature

Two broad satisfaction factors:

- 'Practitioner manner and skill,' which included six core items: practitioner manner, knowledge and competence, general satisfaction, ability to listen and understand, thoroughness and confidentiality/respect for rights
- 'Perceived outcome,' which included: helping relieve symptoms, and maintaining well-being/preventing illness.[4]

Two key criteria (irrespective of medical context):

- Professional competence
- The nature and quality of the patient–health professional relationship.[5]

Factors associated with positive patient satisfaction:

- Patient information provision
- Relationship factors (doctors' friendliness, courteous or encouraging behaviour, social conversation; patients' liking for GP as a person, faith in doctors; partnership building)
- Communication style (for example, patient-centredness, empathy).[6]

These GPs get very little direct feedback from their patients except that 'they keep coming back'. Patients are thought to choose the doctor who suits them best, though this may vary from problem to problem:

'Patients select the listening technique and the doctor of their choice and a lot of it is down to experience and the type and way they wish to be treated. Those who perhaps wish to come for a moan and a groan, take a bit more time, tend to come and see two of us in the partnership and I'm certainly one of those.' (Lew)

There is a feeling that 'People in the community know what sort of doctor you are and will, to a degree, self-select where they go' (Tom) and that 'You get the patients you deserve' (Tim). The patients have been known 'to say "We'll go to the listening doctor"' (Pete), a suggestion supported by Gore and Ogden[7] whose study patients 'actively search out a GP who matches their own representation of the "ideal"'.

It may take a few visits to the surgery to pluck up the courage to discuss a sensitive topic:

'We've all had people who've come in and said, "Actually, I came in and saw Doctor X last week but I couldn't tell him this" and they've been unable to proceed presumably because they didn't hit the right doctor–patient relationship.' (Vic)

'She had been in for a similar consultation with another doctor. I think she had not quite plucked up the courage. She didn't quite get it out that time, so it was a second attempt.' (Phil)

This process may take some time:

'The conversation began, "I've been wanting to tell you about this for about nine months".' (Lew)

Factors associated with patients create pressure and limits on listening. One of these is the content of listening, for example discussion around termination of pregnancy or an illness similar to one presently affecting the GP. Another is the very thick file needing to be studied in depth fully to comprehend the patient's situation. A third is the patient's understanding of the doctor's use of time:

> 'Time is very important to patients. They don't like to be in and out unless they are in a rush themselves. They also don't want to be sitting in the waiting room while you're talking to somebody else about their emotional problems.' (Pat)

It can also be extremely difficult to control or limit listening. In the same way that patients are thought to present cues that demand listening attention in the consultation, there are occasions when the GP feels powerless to limit listening:

> 'I do find it difficult to say "No" and stop consultations. Once people want to pour their heart out to you and they've got stories to tell, they are opening up and giving you an awful lot of their own privacy and their personality and their life and it's a great privilege to sit there and listen to this.' (Adam)

> 'When he comes now, you've sort of resigned yourself to half an hour of listening to his comments (well it seems like half an hour, it may not be). He's a nice chap, you like to listen to him, but if you think he's just prolonging the consultation because he's lonely and just likes to chat, then you are likely to try and draw it to a conclusion.' (Tim)

Despite the availability and use of methods to limit or block listening, enforcing such limits can clearly be problematic. Influences include factors perceived in the patient by the doctor, factors in the content of the listening (such as terminal care) or factors in the doctor (such as discussion of an illness currently affecting the doctor). I discuss the latter, and other factors in the doctor's self, further in Chapters 10 and 11.

In this section, I have described, first, the importance these doctors attribute to listening in their work and, second, the judgements they make within doctor–patient interactions concerning listening. Third, I have described the methods they employ in order not to listen. In the next section, I move on to address relationships, the cumulative consequence of individual doctor–patient interactions.

References

1   Maguire P, Pitceathly C (2002) Key communication skills and how to acquire them. *BMJ.* **325**: 697–700.

2   Rees Lewis J (1994) Patient views on quality care in general practice: literature review. *Soc Sci Med.* **39**: 655–70.

3   Chapple A, Campbell S, Rogers A *et al.* (2002) Users' understanding of medical knowledge in general practice. *Soc Sci Med.* **54**: 1215–24.

4   Greenfield T, Attkisson C (1989) Steps toward a multifactorial satisfaction scale for primary care and mental health services. *Eval Prog Plan.* **12**: 271–8.

5   Williams S, Calnan M (1991) Key determinants of consumer satisfaction with general practice. *Fam Pract.* **8**: 237–42.

6   Williams S, Weinman J, Dale J (1998) Doctor–patient communication and patient satisfaction: a review. *Fam Pract.* **15**: 480–92.

7   Gore J, Ogden J (1998) Developing, validating and consolidating the doctor–patient relationship: the patients' views of a dynamic process. *Br J Gen Pract.* **48**: 1391–4.

Section 2

Listening work and relationships

4

Cumulative listening and relationships

Section 1 focused on the work of listening in the individual GP–patient interaction. This Section concerns doctors' perceptions of the ongoing nature of listening with their patients. This cumulative listening builds relationship between doctor and patient. Chapter 4 presents doctors' perceptions of GP–patient relationships over time and, in Chapter 5, I investigate pastoral work in primary care. Lastly, in Chapters 6 and 7, an example of doctor–patient relationship in primary care (holding) is described and discussed. Holding offers a management tool for a small group of patients who attend regularly without an overt biomedical need.[1]

The day-to-day professional GP–patient interaction in a consultation is the core of the job of the family doctor in primary care. The cumulative effect of such interactions over time builds relationships. These may work well (perhaps with mutual trust and knowledge) or create tensions (if there is, for example, dislike or disagreement). This chapter considers some positive aspects and some difficulties of such relationships.

Involvement and doctor–patient relationship

Words used to describe the positive aspects of GP–patient relationships include *respect, friendliness, empathy, approachability, working through difficult times together, talking in confidence, continuity, intimacy, involvement leading to trust*, and *easy and quick access* to the GP. These GPs feel closer to some of their patients than to others. With some there is 'merely' a working doctor–patient relationship, others the doctor gets to know better. Various factors may influence this; the most important would appear to be simply spending time with people. Getting to know a patient, even in the frailty of an illness and even a patient initially perceived as being 'curmudgeonly' by the GP, affects the relationship and generally increases openness, understanding and mutual respect, which in turn may lead to giving extra time or availability.

At times the doctor may learn more about the patient (or, more rarely, vice versa) and the relationship may change. Descriptive words used include *friendly, comfortable, confidence, trust* and *unique*:

> 'Good background knowledge of the patient and the family' may put the GP 'in a better position to offer advice.' (Rick)

Other relationships are purely working relationships, confined to doctor or patient or medical, and words like *respect, barriers* and *gulf* are used to describe them. Relationships work better when the doctor likes the patient and the patient likes the doctor. It is:

> '... just part of the job that some people like you and want to stay with you.' (Pat)

> 'It's who they like, who they feel they get on with and can talk to.' (Phil)

Several doctors felt humble that, in genuinely wanting to help, they:

> '... often seem to be a deeply appreciated part of their patients' lives.' (Tim)

Knowing the patient is:

> '... about contact with patients and having some empathy, some feel about where they are coming from, where they've been, what's happening to them. It just comes with time. It's what GPs are all about.' (Chaz)

But, knowing may also involve:

> '... a gulf between doctor and patient. There has to be that professional respect both ways. He is a patient and I am his doctor, not necessarily any closer than that.' (Lee)

Similarly, the GP will:

> '... mostly not know them in any great depth. We see people in their frailty. We don't see them in their everyday lives. We know some of their strengths and weaknesses and how they cope with difficulties and so on in a way that's quite a privilege. It's difficult to put into words. They trust us with a lot and they put their confidence in us and we've got a lot of power over them.' (Don)

A longer quote sums up some of these ideas:

'... to know a patient is where the patient comes in to see you and you know all about all the past things that have happened to them. You don't necessarily know all the intimacies of all their personal and social life, but you know why they've come in to see you before. If they come in and complain about their abdomen, you know that they've had irritable bowel in the past and a normal colonoscopy two years ago.

I would mean, by a patient I know, that you don't have to start from scratch with them. You know their family by this stage. You've been in practice for a certain length of time and you know that they're married and how many children they've got and probably how well they get on with their husband and ... you've got their address and you know where they live and so you know more than the average person would know off the street about that particular patient.

A locum sitting in starts completely from scratch, they don't know any of the patients. But when you say that you *know* your patient ... you'll say "How's Jessica, she had the problem a few weeks ago, how's she doing?". So you know about their family, you know about their environment, you know about their past medical history and perhaps some of their past social personal history as well. So that sort of thing really, rather than knowing all the intimate details about their life. I mean you may do if they've told you but not necessarily.

And as regards them knowing you, they don't know you at all. Absolutely nothing at all about you, I don't think. They know how you consult, they know how you interact with them, they know what your reactions are probably going to be to certain situations and they know a bit about your personality but they know nothing about *you* really. But they often feel they do, don't they ...?' (Lee)

Some patients are thought to be more important to their GPs than others in three ways. The first is that 'no one sticks out for any length of time' and 'the only person who is important to me is the patient who walks through the door' for this consultation:

'One could say that they are all important.' (Alex)

Second, rather than importance, which by implication ranks, grades or even judges people, there is the doctor's degree of involvement at any one time:

'I wouldn't have described them as being important to me. They have no more importance to me than any other patients, it's just that I'm more involved with them at that particular time.' (Pete)

'People are important for a while if they've got a critical illness or whatever.' (Pat)

Other examples were patients undergoing special treatments, who were terminally ill, or with an uncertain diagnosis. The key feature of this group of patients for almost all these doctors was that the involvement or importance was 'for a while' or 'at that particular time'.

Third, there are specific patients or groups of patients to whom the word *important* might be applied. The groups include successes, failures and disasters, people who have elicited deep feelings, those whom the GP has got to know, and people with whom the GP has spent time. Three particularly important groups were ex-colleagues, patients known personally to their GPs away from the professional relationship (for example, friends, cleaners, neighbours), and people known to their GPs through many stages of life (for example, children seen from birth to adulthood, young mothers seen from pregnancy to the menopause or retirement). The specific patients generally had major or chronic illness such as cancer, active rheumatoid arthritis, multiple sclerosis or severe congestive cardiac failure. Others mentioned included the manipulative patient, the father figure, the patient who won't see anyone else, the over-appreciative patient, the patient with whom the GP feels a failure, the patient whose life the GP saved, the 'spot diagnosis', the person who helped when the car broke down, the old person with a life story to tell, and the person who previously lived in a particular house.

Long-term doctor–patient relationships

The long-term GP–patient relationship is well recognised and important for the majority of these doctors. It is seen as central to the ethos of family medicine and an invaluable asset in managing patients. Relationships are thought to work better if the patient endeavours always to see the same GP. This continuity is to do with being looked upon as:

'... *their* GP, not just *a* GP. Although they may not want to see you for years, they expect you to know about their father, mother, and grandfather before them or whatever and the ins and outs of everything.' (Tim)

Such long-term knowledge of individuals, their families and their networks is thought to be appreciated by patients, to be very much the unique responsibility of the local GP, and to help in the current doctor–patient relationship:

'You are established and you can remember when Mrs A died and child B was born and so you are very much the family doctor.' (Sam)

As a result, there is increased understanding, trust, insight and openness – relationships become easier to manage, talking is facilitated, problems are anticipated and treatment is more accurately tailored for that specific person.
   The ability to listen seems to become easier as the doctor develops more experience both in life and in general practice:

'As you get to know your patients better, they become more confident of you, you become more confident of them.' (Tim)

The GP of some years standing:

'... is more likely to have established trust between doctor and patient and has a unique insight into life.' (Steve)

It may:

'... take five years as a principal to get the experience in dealing with people' (Matt)

and to build up a global picture of the families in the local community. This may be:

'... easier if you are a parent. You have to listen when you're a parent.' (Alex)

Perhaps the deepest long-term relationships mentioned were those with the bereaved spouse of a patient for whom the GP had managed terminal illness. The bereaved partner is thought to be often reassured by contact with the GP, attending wanting to remember. In this situation, the doctor is perhaps acting as a witness or a significant part of the collective memory of society – I discuss this further in Chapter 12.
   Some long-term relationships present specific challenges, such as limiting the number of investigations performed on a demanding patient (*see* Chapter 7). The disadavantages of the long-term relationship are mentioned in terms of comfort and complacency, resulting in the potential for missed or incorrect diagnoses, and the possibility of incorrectly anticipating problems and dismissing someone before they even enter the room. Similarly, presuming to understand on the basis of previous interactions and jumping to conclusions, or cutting someone short, may sometimes save time but carries

the danger of making incorrect assumptions.

The long-term doctor–patient relationship evolves over the years, and while some continue and flourish, others change for different reasons. There were several reports of patients who stay with a particular GP for many years despite suggestions that they might like to see another doctor and considerable strains, such as arguments with the doctor, rows with practice staff, problems with medication, and the inability of the GP to meet the patient's demands. Other patients do not fall out with their GP but quietly decide to see another doctor; they:

> '... go and you don't know why. Sometimes the ones you've done an awful lot for, kick you hardest.' (Don)

An angry wife may blame the GP for aspects of her late husband's diagnosis and care, despite a long-term relationship, and elect to see another doctor.

Another reason suggested for the breakdown of the long-term doctor–patient relationship is the patient's feeling that they may have let down their GP. They may feel reluctant to discuss, for example, alcoholism in front of someone who has known them very well for many years, perhaps since childhood. It may be easier to start afresh with a clean slate in a relationship that carries less history.

Difficulties in doctor–patient relationships

Aside from these problems of long-term relationships, other examples emerged of difficulties in the doctor–patient relationship. Several doctors have a small group of patients whom they do not like or with whom they find it difficult to sustain a relationship:

> 'You can't like everybody.' (Steve)

There was a general understanding that, given the breadth of human nature, it is part of the GP's role to see:

> '... some people who are just unpleasant, who will mug old grannies, murder, steal cars and all sorts.' (Steve)

The GP will sometimes find certain people unpleasant, unreasonable, stressful, time-wasting or demanding. There are:

'... patients who demand and demand and demand and you know that you can't deliver what they want.' (Phil)

The GP may dread a particular patient attending the surgery and keep that person at arm's length:

'... cringe when their name appears on the list.' (Alex)

It was emphasised that this is a small group of individuals who often lack insight into the effect of their relationship on their doctor and keep returning to the same GP. Such relationships, which may change in nature given time, are accepted as a small but normal part of day-to-day primary care work.
  Patients:

'maybe disagree with what you say, or never do what you tell them.' (Ben)

Or they may be seen as:

'... nowadays far less trusting and far more critical. They come and say things like, "I've looked up my condition on the internet and I want to try this treatment". They know more about the illness then you do!' (Alex)

This is subtly different to the 'demanding' of the previous paragraph. Patients who are willing to challenge their doctor's authority or level of knowledge are seen as demanding in a different way from the patient who is just unpleasant, bad-mannered or rude.
  In some relationships, doctors feel on a treadmill, heavily leant on by their patients and unable to make progress. There is general resignation to the responsibilities and burdens of such patients, who may or may not be labelled 'heartsinks':

'Whatever you do and however much you actually input to that illness, she is not motivated to get out of it and I find her very difficult.' (Phil)

'We've all got our share of those.' (Pete)

'He's going to do it to somebody, it might as well be me. I've sort of resigned myself to the fact.' (Will)

Some patients are seen as angry with the practice or the GP. This anger may be obviously demonstrated and for a specific reason (an example given being blaming the GP who prescribed some medication for the unfortunate side-effects which resulted), or it may be more diffuse, such as general anger for the inadequacies and slowness of NHS referral procedures. Other examples of unexpected animosity towards the GP are being given the blame for hospital treatment that has not worked or being challenged by an irate mother new to the practice with a sick child.

Commonly mentioned was the necessity, from time to time, to be blunt with patients or confront them. This might involve asking a patient to leave the surgery or being firm with a demanding drug addict who claims to have lost a prescription. Being direct or somewhat abrupt was described as a tool in some difficult consultations, to move things on. This is thought to alter the doctor–patient relationship to the extent that the patient may choose to see another doctor in the future or, in contrast, may establish or strengthen the relationship. Perversely, having a row or laying down strong guidelines can cement the relationship, which then becomes long term:

> 'I've only ever fallen out with one patient and she now is back with me and waves at me all the time. That's the only one I've actually said "You shouldn't be here" and had to ask her to leave the surgery. But she was being quite unreasonable, shouting at me literally.' (Pete)

In attempting to persuade someone reluctant to take medication but with an obvious weeping skin infection that needs a few days' antibiotics for a complete cure, Ben describes:

> '... making a choice and deciding that in that consultation I was going to stick to my guns and this was how it was going to be. Not actually so much a two-way communication as being a very old-fashioned directive doctor ... He came back the following week and was loads better.' (Ben)

Other difficulties noted involve the person calling for frequent home visits, the patient who overwhelms the doctor with presents and expects almost 'private' treatment in return (*see* Chapter 9), the man who (consciously or unconsciously) is sexually threatening to the female GP, the patient who overtly wants an affair or the female patient who flamboyantly strips off unnecessarily in front of the male doctor. There is a general feeling that:

> '... in a professional environment, patients as well as doctors should be professional.' (Vic)

Cumulative listening and developing relationships over time are seen as important by these GPs. They are positive about observing families grow up, spending time with people over the years, helping someone through a bad patch and watching them moving on, relating to a young mother who herself was in their care as an infant, and having the privilege of helping someone to a peaceful death who has been their patient for many years. They feel closer to some patients than to others and their degree of involvement varies over time. Some relationships create difficulties which require management – these, and the boundary pressures involved, are discussed further in Section 3. In the remaining chapters of this section, I outline GP–patient relationships in which people attend (sometimes regularly) for support from the doctor without an overt biomedical need.

Reference

1   Cocksedge S, May C (2005) Pastoral and holding work in primary care: affect, subjectivity and chronicity. *Chronic Illness.* **1**(2): 153–9.

5

Pastoral work in primary care

The role of the listening GP

Part of the role of the listening GP is to get:

'... involved in their lives; they trust you, most of them anyway.' (Alex)

Some of this is about availability and accessibility, and the fact that going to see the doctor is a socially acceptable thing to do. Also important is the confidentiality of the family doctor and just being there for the patient:

'People come because they're not quite sure where to go and talk to somebody in confidence about things, particularly of a personal nature.' (Tim)

'He was just using me as a sounding board, just talking through his problems. I was there just as someone to talk to and to listen. He wasn't after an answer, he was just after talking really.' (Pete)

Additionally, this listening role may involve being there to legitimate and validate people's experience, to let them touch base and check with someone (I discuss this further in Chapter 12):

'They came in with a problem with their daughter, not a clinical problem. They seemed to find it helpful to hear that I see other mothers in the same situation as them and they are not alone in that. It was obviously such a weight off her mind that other people's daughters did similar things and that it was often just a one-off and didn't really lead to anything else. That particular consultation was very rewarding, just as rewarding as perhaps diagnosing hypertension.' (Jo)

'People say, "I've never talked to anyone about this before doctor," and I feel so humble really.' (Pat)

Such listening work, which I have called pastoral work, is thought to suit the GP who is:

'... more interested in people and the way they present their problems than the actual disease process.' (Chris)

'Everybody can get some comfort in coming. We may not be the world's greatest clinician but they hopefully can go out and say "Well at least I was able to say my bit".' (Tim)

The doctor needs:

'... a genuine willingness or almost enjoyment in involving oneself in other people's lives, emotions and feelings, and actually not being afraid to do that.' (Lew)

In contrast, while accepting listening as part of their work, some are constantly looking for the rare diagnosis that comes along every year or two:

'The consultation I like is where someone comes in with something trivial and you turn up something which is going to alter their life, like aortic aneurysm or meningococcal meningitis. I like doing clever diagnosis, I'm sure any doctor does. I don't mind listening but they are not the most fulfilling consultations. Problem consultations are when I think someone's ill and I don't know what's going on.' (Pete)

'I get really excited when somebody comes in with a brilliant clinical sign and you get it all sorted out. I get quite high about that because it doesn't happen very often. Being a good listener doesn't give me the same adrenaline rush, but it's a whole different ball game and I do enjoy the listening consultations.' (Lee)

Nevertheless, listening, either in a single interaction or as part of an ongoing relationship, is central to the work of these GPs and is required much more often than 'clever diagnoses'. The role of the GP in listening work is as much about subjective, psychosocial issues (such as being a sounding board) as about biomedical and objective clinical pathology.

Descriptions of pastoral listening work

A variety of descriptions of the meaning of pastoral work in primary care emerged. There was general agreement that being pastoral involves being supportive, caring, empathic and reassuring, and does not usually involve clinical medicine. It could include acting as someone to talk to while a life event is gradually worked through or being a shoulder to cry on. It is about lending an ear, being used as another responsible adult or a sounding board, perhaps offering guidance or:

> '... arm over the shoulder good friendly advice.' (Lew)

It may entail sharing some of life's experiences or giving an opinion. It could involve:

> '... helping people to make their own decisions.' (Chaz)

> '... rubber stamping a course of action.' (Matt)

Phrases such as 'common sense fatherly/motherly advice' (Sam) are used several times. The following quotation seems to sum up several of these descriptions:

> 'The role of the family doctor in these situations is just supporting really, just being available, just being there in a fragmented world, showing that you are there when they need you, an outlet for their feelings really, just understanding them and what they are going through and showing empathy, hand holding (metaphorically speaking) ...' (Phil)

There is also a recognition that, although the word *pastoral* may have religious or ecclesiastic connotations for some people, pastoral work in primary care, as described in this chapter, is a central and essential part of the GP's job and does not imply any specific religious or spiritual awareness or input by the doctor.

The definition which emerged of being pastoral was 'being available for reliable supportive care not concerned with clinical medicine'. It does not include those consultations that are purely administrative, such as filling out a passport form or an insurance claim.

Examples of pastoral work

Examples of pastoral problems brought to the GP are numerous and include relationship or marital problems, stress, worry, 'things at home', lifestyle issues, bereavement:

> 'How they've conducted themselves or how somebody's related to them' (Tom)

or people:

> '... who can't cope with life or have inappropriate expectations of life' (Sam)

teenagers who fall out with their parents (and vice versa), elderly relatives, women overwhelmed by the burdens of family life, people who are marginalised or knocked down, redundancy, children and their families with problems at school, issues within families, 'time of life' difficulties, social issues or difficulties with neighbours. Clearly, this list is incomplete but it gives an idea of the breadth of pastoral work that may be brought into the consulting room. It can be summarised as:

- family and relationship issues
- loss and bereavement
- lifestyle and social issues
- other life events.

Advocacy and liaison are also part of the role of the GP in pastoral work. There is a general understanding that:

> 'It's easier to come to the doctor than to whatever other agency.' (Vic)

> 'Pastoral care is what the vicar should be doing but patients tend to come to the doctor nowadays.' (Vic)

It does not *have* to be the GP who responds to this cry for help from this patient – members of other professional or voluntary organisations may be better trained to help, and pointing people in the right direction or putting them in touch with other helpers is a legitimate function for the GP. Possibilities include volunteer organisations, such as CRUSE for bereavement, the Citizens Advice Bureau and other advice centres, and other professionals, such as clergy, social services, mental health teams including community psychiatric nurses, occupational and disability advisors and the legal profession. Feelings are mixed as to whether some of these agencies can fill the place of the GP adequately, particularly given their lack of continuity of personnel sometimes. It is also important, given:

> '... the great and nebulous variety of things that we are asked, to be careful to give impartial advice and say "Look I'm not an expert at this"' (Rick)

particularly where financial or legal affairs are concerned.

Doctors' views on pastoral work

Although pastoral work had not been given much thought by these GPs, their views are generally along the lines of:

'It is appropriate and I'm happy to do it.' (Will)

It is seen as a core part of the job and there is an appreciation that many, if not most, consultations have a pastoral element. There is an understanding that, while the issues considered may not be clinical medicine and although it is not essential to be a doctor to be of assistance, this person has chosen this time to consult their family doctor about an issue that is of importance to them and thus it has to be an appropriate and reasonable part of the role of the GP:

'I am very happy to be here as a friend within the professional relationship' (Paul)

and with all the background knowledge of the experienced GP. Although there was a strong consensus that pastoral work is part of the job:

'It's what we are there for' (Phil)

one doctor argued that:

'It's not the best use of our time – it's very time-consuming and old-fashioned.' (Pete)

Another commented that:

'I think patients feel it's very valuable but a lot of doctors think they're wasting their time.' (Matt)

The words used in describing why people expect their GP to be pastoral include *reliability, safety, permanence, normality, continuity, trust, respect, friendship, professionalism, easy access, no cost,* and *social acceptability*. Seeing the GP is:

'. . . just part of life' (Pat)

and often:

'There is no one else to talk to.' (Steve)

With the reduction in extended families, where someone might have talked to grandma or the priest in the past, the GP may instead provide 'a sort of elder', 'another family', with whom there is an ongoing relationship.

It is thought to be easier to take on a pastoral role when, as a GP:

> ' … you are a bit older with a few more grey hairs' (Lew)

having had your own family, and with perhaps:

> '… some wisdom and authority from having been in this game a few years.' (Lew)

Pastoral work occurs more frequently as the GP gets older and has been in practice longer. There are no rules or guidelines concerning this role:

> 'You do what you think is right. I suppose I have learnt some of it from my mother.' (Sam)

Sometimes this extends to feeling the need to be quite sharp with someone, to 'name' an issue, to actively encourage someone or overtly give them permission for a certain course of action, or even to tell them off.

Difficulties in pastoral work

The most frequent difficulty was the perceived threat of a general anti-professionalism currently present in society reducing patients' confidence in their GP:

> 'When you lose those sort of people to talk to that you have confidence in, where do you go? I don't know what you do.' (Ben)

Similarly, organisational changes in the health service are thought to both put increasing time pressures on the GP, and question the whole concept of the family doctor with an established relationship and background knowledge of the patient and family, which may result in pastoral work being squeezed out.

Fears about pastoral work are mostly concerned with the possibility of being overwhelmed by demand (though with an acknowledgement that in practice this does not occur) and feeling inadequately equipped because of the lack of any formal training:

> 'Initially you wonder whether you're capable of coping with that, whether you really have got the knowledge or the experience. But when you do

come to a conclusion and you see something working, you feel rather chuffed by it. You think, "Well yes that was quite useful and probably more useful that just taking somebody's blood pressure for the sixth time that year" or whatever.' (Tim)

Another fear was of getting the right balance between giving opinionated, certain, dogmatic, didactic or paternalistic advice and enabling someone to reach their own conclusion in their own way:

'I never know whether I'm supposed to be helping them by giving them solutions or letting them explore, because it's quite easy for some of us to say, "Well this is what you should do". That is not what you are there for, but sometimes that's what they want. "What do you think I should do, doctor?" I don't know ... what are the answers?' (Phil)

In conclusion, it is apparent from this analysis that pastoral work in the doctor–patient encounter (defined as 'being available for reliable supportive care not concerned with clinical medicine') is seen as a frequently occurring core part of listening work in primary care, which some doctors feel poorly equipped to undertake. It may occur in a single interaction or as part of an ongoing relationship. Pastoral work is about psychosocial issues and subjective pathology, and may involve validation or legitimation of a patient's experience. Some of these issues are further discussed in Chapter 7 and in Section 3.

6

Holding work: description

In the next two chapters, I present an example of a GP–patient relationship: holding. 'Holding' is concerned with 'being there' for the patient, 'keeping them going' at a variety of different levels and possibly reducing their demands overall on the service. These doctors report widespread holding going on every day in GPs' surgeries. In this chapter, I describe the properties of holding work and outline some factors in its use. In Chapter 7, I discuss the value of holding and consider other related issues.

The concept of holding

Holding work was immediately recognised and readily identified by the vast majority of these doctors as a routine part of everyday primary care. The definition which emerged was of work aimed at 'establishing and maintaining a trusting, constant, reliable GP–patient relationship that is concerned, not with cure, but with support, giving time and keeping people going'. It provides ongoing and reliable support to which people can return:

'Someone they trust being there if and when needed, which keeps them "ticking over".' (Paul)

The sorts of phrases and words that were used to describe the concept of holding included:

'You often end up being the one they come back to.' (Ben)

'There are some people, I agree, who at the end of the day you end up having to be there for and maintain.' (Rick)

'The amount of support they need is fairly small. It's just someone they know they can rely on. Someone in authority, someone who, I think, they have respect for. Just to know that that person is concerned about them, I think, gives them quite a lot of benefit and reassurance.' (Huw)

'To some extent it's probably a constancy. The fact that we're there. They know they can trust you, if they know they've got something to fall back on.' (Don)

The group of patients being held by any single GP with an average list at any one time was small, up to 20 people from all age groups over the age of 20 years. Overall, there was a strong consensus in the accounts that the concept of holding people by GPs is helpful because:

'It's better to see them more frequently and know what's going on.' (Don)

A very small minority of these doctors either did not recognise the concept of holding in their patients or recognised the concept but actively tried to avoid undertaking any holding for their patients.

Types of holding

Three types of holding emerged: long-term holding, either continuous or episodic, and interim holding.

Continuous long-term holding

This was recognised by almost every GP:

'A patient who comes in every two months or so ... I feel like I'm a moral support and just an outlet for her really. It seems to help support her. I feel quite sorry for her. ... I referred her to the counsellor but she ends up coming back to me at the end of the day. I've seen her for two years now and I'll probably carry on seeing her. I think it's been vital for her and it has helped her.' (Phil)

Typically, these patients have had an acute episode (such as a physical illness or a life event which may or may not have required treatment), but they do not have current physical problems. Continuous long-term holding has evolved after completion of the acute episode and supports the patient. Often other members of the primary care team have been involved in caring for these patients for a while, but after that their long-term care reverts to their GP.

Similar comments further describe doctors' perceptions of the therapeutic nature of long-term holding:

'Seeing him regularly about every two months for a period of several years seemed to keep him ticking over. It kept the situation stable.' (Paul)

'She was widowed about four years ago and was very isolated after his death. I just say, "Pop in to see me about once every four months". There's not a lot medically I can do for her except let her get it off her chest.' (Huw)

'It's a very small group but I think they do have to come. It does give them a lift just to keep them on the straight and narrow for another month or two.' (Vic)

Continuous long-term holding involves seeing people regularly over a period of years. From a purely medical point of view, this regular attendance involves little in the way of active treatment or investigation. However, it is thought to provide reassurance and support, and to be therapeutic in keeping people going or 'ticking over'.

Episodic long-term holding

This involves patterned clinical encounters over a period of months or years, a series of episodes of holding within the context of a long-term relationship:

'You would be holding them for a bit and then it would peter out and they might then be back to see you in a few months or a year later when something else happens.' (Huw)

Interim holding

This falls between routine general practice and long-term holding. In the former, a person may be seen for a few appointments while an episode of illness is negotiated. For example, someone with a chest infection might be seen two or three times for initial diagnosis, treatment and follow-up. Long-term holding is a much longer relationship, lasting years rather than months. Interim holding emerges between these two as a regular doctor–patient interaction which lasts a few months or so, but generally not more than 12 months:

'These patients I think suddenly come to a head, burn themselves out and disappear again. ... They would come with these enormous worries and problems. You would find it very difficult to live with all the problems that they pour out to you, and for a while there's nothing you can do apart from listen. And suddenly, they've gone, they disappear. So these problems come to a head and burn themselves out. For a while you're very much involved and have to see them regularly. I would be quite happy to see them three times a week in the initial stages because if there's nothing else you can do, at least you can see them again and talk to them.' (Steve)

Someone in this group would see their GP regularly for between a few weeks and a few months. Regularly might mean weekly initially, moving to monthly or bimonthly as necessary. The doctor offers support, reassurance and a listening ear, along with medication as appropriate. Interim holding is clearly identified as a normal part of everyday general practice by these doctors.

Reasons for holding

The main reasons for holding were mental health problems (non-acute, non-psychotic), loss and bereavement, and relationship difficulties.

Patients with mental health problems, or a past history of such problems, are the most commonly mentioned group of those needing holding. The largest group in this category are those with long-term mild depression or those who have had depression in the past but are thought to be helped by keeping in touch with the doctor:

'They've had depression in the past and we've maybe got them off the tablets or some of them are still on the tablets. But again, they seem to need to come down every four to eight weeks when they are fine, trekking along fine. They feel the need to come and again, one wonders why.' (Vic)

Other groups mentioned by one or two doctors as possibilities for holding are anxiety (short-term and chronic), alcohol dependency, post-natal depression, borderline or inadequate personalities, bipolar disorder and anorexia nervosa.

Another main group in this category are those patients who have been bereaved. Often, the GP has been intimately involved in the death of the spouse and may be one of the few people who still remembers the partner, providing a link with the past. Those doctors perceive that such patients wish to be held and supported:

'The ones that spring to mind are those where I have been involved in the bereavement, the death of their partners. That's a big group and certainly involves holding. One shares very intimate moments with them and they keep on coming back and wanting to perhaps remember those moments.' (Adam)

'She built up the relationship with me as his doctor and when he died, she looked to me. There's nobody else for her to talk to and I think she links me with him. . . . Basically just supporting her every couple of months.' (Ed)

Relationship problems form another large category in this group:

'. . . keeping in touch maybe every two or three months to see that they are on top of things. They may not actually say much when they come in. I've been seeing one young woman for some years. Men have not been good to her and she's had a lot of psychological problems. She just needs to come in and see where she's at.' (Don)

Other life problems, such as financial difficulties, stress and generally not coping, are also mentioned.

By far the most common problem associated with interim holding was working through a major life event, such as the break-up of a marriage or depression:

'I think if people have a life event going on, like a marital split-up, you can do a supportive role. This is a temporary problem and, although it seems awful, it will sort itself out one way or the other and it won't be the end of life as we know it. Reassurance and trying to keep people off benzodiazepines with occasional use of antidepressants if they seem appropriate. Try and give them a bit of support and reassurance that they are not going barmy while the life event is gradually worked through.' (Ben)

'There will be phases when you feel as if you're holding the depressives. They either recover or you'll pass them on. So they're a transient crowd but they could be with you for six to twelve months.' (Sam)

This interim holding has the clear clinical objective of seeing the patient regularly to contain the situation while the patient 'works through' the event, allowing minimum use of pharmacological treatment.

There was also a recognition that chronic medical problems (generally mild) may be used as an excuse to see the doctor and to maintain a holding relationship:

'She's got mild hypertension, very well controlled, and glaucoma. She goes to the eye clinic. There's probably no real medical reason for me to see her but she is very isolated. I'm not actually diagnosing, not necessarily prescribing. She just comes and unloads and I check her BP and off she goes again.' (Huw)

'I've been seeing him regularly since she died. He's had some skin problems and a minor leg ulcer but I think the benefit of the consultations is a quick look at those and then we sit and talk about nothing in particular.' (Tim)

Similarly, some patients have had chronic medical problems in the past and still feel the need to see the doctor occasionally:

'There are people who have had medical problems that now aren't active, and very much need just to come every so often and be listened to. I feel it is important to do that and I don't have a problem with that. ... She had a stroke some years ago and was left with a severe degree of dysphasia. She lost her job because of this and is divorced. She just has a need to come in every month or so and have her 10 minutes.' (Chris)

There was a distinction between people with largely psychosocial problems needing a holding relationship and people with physical or organic illness needing ongoing monitoring activities, such as hypertension or on hormone replacement therapy, which might well be delegated to practice nurses. Similarly, those with other chronic conditions having more immediate and practical medical needs (such as multiple sclerosis and cancer) are thought to require a 'key worker' or co-ordinator role from the doctor.

Managing holding

Holding may be led by the doctor or led by the patient and it may be agreed in advance or occur *de facto*. If the holding is doctor led:

'It's very much doctor led. You're saying "I want to see you every six months" and she's saying, "Oh all right then".' (Rick)

Reasons for leading holding include reducing patients' worry, regulating frequency of attendance, trying to ensure regular attendance and anticipating or pre-empting problems:

'I normally say to people, "I would like to see you in two months". If you don't do that, my belief is that they worry about whether they should come or they shouldn't come.' (Will)

'I usually say, "I think we'd better check this again in a month" or whatever. If I didn't suggest this, he'd be back in a week.' (Tim)

'I see her about once a month and she would try and see me more often, but I can say, "Look I only saw you the other day, I know this situation". So I control it that way.' (Huw)

'I try and encourage her to come regularly because, every so often, she will miss an appointment and you won't see her for a while and then she will come back in quite a state really. ... Once a month is fine and it is usually quite a quick appointment. She seems to do better ticking over because she is such hard work when she actually starts again.' (Jo)

'I think it is better to see them more frequently and know what's going on and respond to crises if they arise. If they know that they can come and talk to you, they can trust you and they know they've got something to fall back on.' (Don)

'There's almost a feeling that you are capturing the symptoms with some people, getting ahead of the game a little bit. I feel that I'm seeing them every now and again, just before I think they go off. It keeps them ticking over really.' (Ben)

Management of holding varies from doctor to doctor and from patient to patient, and will be influenced by how well the doctor knows the patient. In managing holding, some doctors are quite forceful, whereas others are quite clear that holding is patient led; some feel obliged to see people regularly, whereas others are much firmer about their boundaries:

'Every time she comes to see me, she wants to know when she's got to come again. So you feel duty bound to say "OK, come again next month," and off she goes quite happy.' (Steve)

'She runs that. I have often thought I should tackle it and I haven't done. I don't like confronting people and I tend to shy away from addressing things like that.' (Chris)

'I won't say to them, "Look I'll see you in eight weeks' time". I leave it up to them but they don't come back very frequently. So they are in control of the frequency.' (Lee)

' "This is the way we do it and if you behave yourself, I'll carry on looking after you in this way" and it seems to be an agreed arrangement.' (Huw)

'I make it clear, "This is what I can offer you. If you're going to come and see me, these are the ground rules: I can give you this amount of time, however often, and take it or leave it". So you have to be boss, you have to manage that time.' (Rick)

Some people are held by the GP while also seeing other health professionals, often the mental health team or the practice counsellor. The GP is thought to provide aspects of care that these patients do not find elsewhere:

'She still sees the psychiatrist every six months and the community psychiatric nurse every two weeks. She comes in to have a chat about all the symptoms and her worries. Most of the time I just nod my head. It's more really like a friend, like someone to unload her problems to, and there's no answer to them.' (Matt)

Although other members of the primary care team may be involved in caring for these patients for a while, ultimately their long-term care reverts to their GP, who is contractually obliged to continue caring work. These doctors accept this as part of their work, their only permanent method of ending the relationship being removal of the patient from their list.

Problems with holding

A variety of problems associated with holding have been identified. The first and most common point concerns the doctor's capacity to acknowledge that holding may be valid and useful, that:

'Keeping them on the straight and narrow for another month is not wasting my time' (Vic)

without getting frustrated by lack of apparent progress. Some doctors:

'... struggle to see the value' (Will)

of holding their patients, and it may be hard for the GP to accept the importance of holding as a role:

'They obviously see it as quite a major crutch to their life. We perhaps don't realise how important it is.' (Phil)

'You've got to learn not to reach for the prescription pad and be satisfied just to talk to them.' (Sam)

'I try to dissuade people from latching on to me – I think I've got more to offer people over a period of illness that has a beginning and an end.' (Ed)

Those doctors who are prepared to take on a holding relationship have feelings about their patients in this group which include frustration, irritation and inadequacy. Fears in taking on the holding role centre on feelings of impotence, uselessness and being weighed down:

'I feel as though I'm shouldering a burden the practice has.' (Chaz)

'She's quite frustrating. I feel useless really and it doesn't seem to serve any purpose, apart from someone perhaps keeping a vague eye on her.' (Pete)

There was a particular concern that patients might pick up these feelings in some way from their doctors. If holding is acknowledged and named as a purposive and normal part of work, some of these feelings may be reduced.
    The process of establishing a holding relationship with a particular patient can be problematic as a switch is made from the normal medical model of diagnosis and treatment to the holding model:

'I think the phase of coming to terms with that holding policy can be quite stressful for doctors but once the arrangement is reached, it is actually not as demanding.' (Lew)

Part of this phase is the ability to confront and alter the expectations of both patient and doctor, accepting that:

'Some problems aren't amenable to much at all.' (Ben)

Lack of skills was noted by a few doctors, both in establishing and then maintaining an ongoing holding relationship. As doctors differ in their normal consulting styles, it seems likely they will also differ in their holding styles, and that:

'Different partners will have different numbers of patients like that.' (Adam)

'When those consulters who do the five-minute, bang bang, in–out consultations are away for a bit, I see their patients and I think they use different means than I would use. What I've found quite interesting is that the holding mechanism and method seems to be more doctor dependent than patient dependent. I can think of one patient who comes in to see my partner and has a very brief five-minute consultation, bang bang. When they come to see me, it's more likely to be 10 or 15 minutes … So I suspect my abilities for holding are focused more around listening interaction rather than, "Right that's it, you've had your slot and off you go". It does raise the worry that my holding abilities might not actually be as cost effective as somebody else's.' (Lew)

The possibility that one doctor might become the 'holding doctor' for the practice was also mentioned as a worry by a doctor who occasionally receives referrals from his partners of patients needing a holding relationship.

The general fear about pressure of time discussed earlier is also a concern for holding work. However, the time needed for holding can be managed:

'I now know how long they're going to take before they come usually' (Steve)

and these patients form a small proportion of the average GP's workload:

'If there was a lot, I would feel bad about it because of pressure of time and appointments. But it is a minority.' (Vic)

Indeed, some doctors found themselves, once in a holding relationship:

'… not being frightened or worrying about the workload that these people create but feeling more happy to take responsibility to follow these problems through.' (Will)

Inappropriate holding

There is a small but significant subgroup which I have called inappropriate holding. It contains three categories in which continued holding may be unhelpful to either patient or doctor.

The first category of inappropriate holding involves patients who see the GP as the only one who can solve their problems:

'There are one or two patients who certainly treat me in an unrealistically reverent way. It is a nice feeling in some respects but dangerous too.' (Lew)

'I've learnt over the years that there are certain people who will monopolise your time because they think you're the only one that can do it. I think that's a self-delusion. It makes you feel good at first when somebody thinks only you can do the business but I don't agree with it basically.' (Rick)

This could also work in the opposite direction, with GPs seeing themselves as the only ones who can solve all their patient's problems. 'Monopolising' the doctor's time suggests inappropriate or frequent attendance at the surgery requiring management – I discuss this further in the next chapter.

Secondly, GPs out of their depth in a therapeutic situation will help neither themselves nor their patients:

'I saw one person, who had a very difficult childhood, weekly for months and months and months, and we didn't get anywhere at all really. It was very difficult. There were lots of self-harm attempts and para-suicides and I just felt I needed to keep on meeting. I used to give long appointments and they would always run to about half an hour and that was very tiring. ... I think I am wary that I don't want to get into that situation again.' (Jo)

The report given of this relationship suggests that the doctor may have underestimated the boundaries and limits of therapeutic competence and strayed inadvertently into the field of the psychotherapist. Such unrecognised straying could have negative consequences for the patient, the GP and the long-term doctor–patient relationship. Part of the GP's skill must be firstly in identifying boundaries and requesting help when needed. Second, GPs need to be aware of colleagues from other disciplines locally (such as counselling, psychotherapy or psychiatry) who can be approached for advice, support or referral if necessary.

The last category of inappropriate holding involves legitimate but unmanageable holding. In this situation, long-term holding is appropriate but the GP and the patient are unable to manage the situation effectively to make it work:

'[Long-term holding] is not terribly onerous. I only see them probably once a month or so. The worst one I ever had, I tried agreements with her but she used to call once or twice a week and it got to the stage where I knew exactly what she was going to say. I put up with that for about a year and a half and then I suggested another doctor went to see her.' (Pete)

In this chapter, I have described holding work in primary care, a significant if small part of listening work in day-to-day practice. These GPs have a group of patients who need to attend regularly and their attending requires managing. Holding work is a method of management for this group, who are thought to need a non-curative, walking-alongside relationship. It would seem to be a specific, but as yet unnamed, function for 'the most frequently used drug in general practice', the doctor him- or herself.[1]

Reference

1   Balint M (1963) *The Doctor, His Patient and the Illness* (2e). Churchill Livingstone, London.

7

Holding work: discussion

Holding work in clinical encounters may be thought of in three ways.

- As a concept: a way of understanding some aspects of GP–patient relationships, a type of person-centred therapeutic alliance.
- As a specific relationship: a way of describing individual GP–patient interactions, which may be either interim or long term.
- As a method of management in listening work: a way of managing some problematic GP–patient encounters.

In this chapter, I discuss dependency and the value of holding work in primary care before presenting some theoretical issues concerning holding.

Dependency and holding

There is an overlap between holding and dependency with a variety of types of dependence described. Two extreme examples of dependence are:

'I think the threat in that situation would be if I felt there was some sort of emotional attachment building to me in an inappropriate way.' (Tom)

'The "little old lady dependency". The lady in her late seventies, in perhaps slightly failing health, still chirpy and wishing to bring you a pot of jam and enquire about your children and comment on your pictures and to bring a couple of minor complaints.' (Lew)

In between is the 'dependent personality':

'It may be unrealistic to try and convert what is a dependent personality into an independent personality. That's their fabric and make-up and that's going to be difficult to change.' (Ben)

Dependency in the doctor–patient relationship may be, first, inappropriate, slightly threatening and unwanted but inevitable because of the vagaries of human nature and personality, or, second, 'little old lady' benign, to be smiled upon as part of the social fabric of primary care work in the community:

> 'There is an element of doctor dependency and in some ways it's flattering, isn't it, but it wears off quite quickly. There is a group of those and usually I'll know them reasonably well and be happy in their management. They tend to be more the elderly groups so I don't find that a problem. If it's "I want to see you doc, I don't want to see anyone else", that's fine.' (Pete)

Third, dependency on the GP may be acceptable, if time-wasting:

> 'A lot of patients are dependent. It's simple things, isn't it, even like management of blood pressure. Try as hard as one might to get them to come back and just have their blood pressure measured by the nurse, they come back to you time and time again. But in itself that's OK. It might be a waste of my time, but it allows me to relax a bit and it's important to have some consultations that aren't too involved, aren't too deep. So I suppose you try and suggest they come back or reduce the frequency of attendance but don't get too angry when they keep on turning up.' (Adam)

There was also a distinction made between the 'little old lady' gentle social dependency in the doctor–patient relationship (and hence not holding) and a therapeutic holding in which a patient is kept stable over a period of time.

> 'It is holding and I don't think that they necessarily have to be dependent. All they are saying is, "Look, you have been a party to my innermost problems and it helped me at the time. Thank you and I would just like to be able, every so often, to check base with you, and let you know how I am getting on" and I mean I'd encourage people to do that, I think. ... It's dependency when I get this sense that they need to come in, come what may, you know, that they actually can't keep away. The dependent people would very rarely come and say, "I'm fine at the moment. While I am here there are three really trivial things, can I ask you about those? But I did just want to tell you that I am OK". Those people are not dependent, whereas the dependent ones come in and are almost kind of fishing around for things to validate their presence in the surgery, and you know they are.' (Chris)

Holding is positive, trusting and potentially therapeutic, with the GP providing support, a reliable base from which to check out, and an ongoing relationship founded on previous interactions. Dependence is, first, inappropriate and possibly threatening, second, gentle, social and benign or, third, time-wasting but acceptable. Additionally, rather than being held by their doctor, some (dependent) patients may 'hold on to' (Adam) their GP, mostly inappropriately. The attitude of the GP towards dependency defines how much these patients are perceived as a problem. Although some doctors are happy to accept dependency at least part of the time, others:

'... firmly wean them off – it is important to manage your time' (Jo)

or worry that they:

'... are not ruthless enough' (Phil)

and that they:

'... foster dependency.' (Chris)

The value of holding within the doctor–patient relationship reflects the boundary between holding and dependence. Someone who is dependent is said to 'depend on another for support', to be 'reliant' or to have 'confident trust'.[1] Holding, as discussed earlier, is thought to be a positive and therapeutic doctor–patient relationship, because keeping someone stable ('ticking over') rather than actively working to alter or improve their condition may be a therapeutic act in itself. Dependence, in the context of the doctor–patient encounter, is either social, benign and appropriate or less positive, inappropriate and perhaps threatening. Dependency is, in part, determined in the doctor's attitude to the individual.

The value of holding

Holding occurs within a trusting confidential doctor–patient relationship:

'They turn to the doctor really, it's just someone they know they can rely on. Someone in authority, someone who they have respect for. Just to know that that person is concerned about them, I think, gives them quite a lot of benefit and reassurance.' (Huw)

Within that relationship, holding challenges the assumption that the role of the doctor is either to cure people or, failing that, to move them forwards:

'Medically and logically I'm doing little for them.' (Lew)

'They tend to have problems where there aren't ultimately any easy solutions.' (Rick)

So the value of holding work is in constant relationships, being there without necessarily making better and simply giving people time, which may keep them going:

'For some people, you end up just having to be there.' (Rick)

'It must give people a bit more worth.' (Pat)

'I feel like I'm a moral support and an outlet for her.' (Phil)

'I was the only person in the end prepared to give him any time. I would be there for him and we would touch base on a regular basis.' (Will)

'I'm keeping him going it seems, keeping the family together.' (Chaz)

The weight of expectations from patients is a burden for some GPs, particularly from those patients who are seen as difficult or heartsink:

'People come and they expect you to solve everything, social, domestic, marital, everything.' (Matt)

Naming holding and engaging in the listening work of establishing a holding relationship with such patients may be functional, positive and valuable:

'She's one of these groan-heartsink patients. I cringe every time I see her name on the list – she's one of my cringe patients.' (Alex)

'They become less of a problem. They just become part of your routine and you accommodate them and adjust for them and don't let it worry you like it used to. It gives patients greater confidence in you if they know that you are happy to see them again.' (Will)

Managing these problem patients by viewing them as in need of a holding relationship accords with the experience of the vast majority of these doctors.

Lastly, the holding relationship is valuable if the doctor has the confidence to hold the patient in primary care and resist demands (from both the patient and their own biomedical training) for referral to hospital and investigations:

'The same symptoms have had extensive investigation for eight or nine years. I finally found a reasonable role as an ongoing damage limitation exercise. I see her about once a month and I eventually decided to provide continuing support and say, "I'm not going to authorise more investigations, even though we may disagree about this". I've now become comfortable with that having found it for years a bit of a drain. Having finally reached my position that I can take this no further, I've accepted that I have a low-level therapeutic role which is actually continuing to support her in a state of relative health despite her own perceptions. If my use is to avoid her disturbing other practitioners and going through the same hoops again while causing herself distress and spending NHS money, then I think it is probably a good investment of my time.' (Lew)

The value of the listening work of holding is in establishing and maintaining a trusting, constant, reliable GP–patient relationship that is concerned not with cure but with support, giving time and keeping people going. Additionally, it may be that simply giving time allows people space in which to gradually improve or grow (*see* 'Holding and attachment' later in this chapter).

The perceptions of these GPs of their own position and value in a holding relationship are of interest:

'There was nobody else around that she felt safe talking to. She felt everybody else was a threat, perhaps too judgemental about the situation.' (Phil)

'Some doctors think "I'm a treatment, seeing me", but I think it's very difficult to actually quantify whether that's true or not.' (Ed)

'Your role is simply to reassure him every time you see him.' (Ben)

'People need to come back at intervals to check on how they are doing. Even if it is brief, to say, "I'm OK" to someone who knows what has gone on.' (Chris)

'It's really like a friend, someone who she'd come to, to unload her problems and there's no answer to them.' (Matt)

'I think that she needs to come in and absolve herself, confess to me.' (Adam)

The doctor as treatment, as friend, as confessor, as safe and non-judgemental, as advisor on perceptions of well-being, as reassurer, as listener able to give time which may feel productive or unproductive — all these are possible roles. In addition, as I have discussed, the GP may be the link with the past when people have been bereaved, or the 'holder of the story' (*see* Chapter 12). Relationships in general practice alter as they become more long term and part of the value of holding is in maintaining continuity in a trusting, reliable relationship:

> 'Constancy, the fact that we're there (and people in the community team come and go). We are someone familiar and we remember what happened to them 10 years ago.' (Don)

> 'I've known some of these people for 20 years and you tend to get mixed up and involved with their lives. I suppose they trust you, most of them anyway.' (Alex)

I discuss holding and trust further later in this chapter. It is hard to estimate the value of holding and of the support provided by the doctor for the patient in trusting, holding relationships. Several epidemiological studies have shown that social and emotional support can protect against premature mortality, prevent illness and aid recovery, and also that emotional distress causes susceptibility to illness.[2–4] It seems reasonable to assume, although this is only an assumption, that at the least holding is doing no harm, even if it is using the GP's time. At best, holding may provide adequate support for the patient to reduce both other illnesses and the necessity for further medical investigations or treatment. This would seem to be a reasonable task for the GP, and these doctors give significant support to individuals, which is often demanding for the doctor. Although doctors may be more satisfied with curing physical problems, keeping someone going by seeing them regularly may also be an achievement.

There is a body of thought in the literature of psychotherapy in which holding clients in a relationship is both central and therapeutic. This may be holding and supporting someone either to allow them to maintain their current level ('ticking over') or to allow them space to work through issues and move on — I discuss this in 'Holding and attachment' later in this chapter. These doctors did not wish to be seen as amateur counsellors. Holding in the general practice context does not appear to require the skills of psychotherapists or counsellors as it is already being used (although not named or valued) in everyday practice.

Holding may be of particular value for patients in certain problematic illness categories in primary care, such as frequent attenders and heartsink patients. It may be helpful to use the holding concept to review, or perhaps rename, some of these problematic GP–patient relationships, with the possibility of reducing the negative stereotyping inherent in, for example, the word *heartsink*. Naming, acknowledging and understanding this process of holding may allow these relationships to be seen in a different light. I discuss this in the penultimate section of this chapter.

Holding and trust

Trust is fundamental to interpersonal relating and community living. In general, individuals relate to others on the assumption that they 'are who they purport to be, will act in accordance with generally assumed norms of behaviour, and will meet their role obligations'.[5] Trust, in interactions outside families or close social networks, is built slowly over time. 'Successful relationships between doctors and patients depend on trust.'[6] In the GP–patient relationship, the patient needs to trust the doctor and the doctor reciprocally to trust the patient.[7] Balint described a 'mutual investment company':

> It is on this basis of mutual satisfaction and mutual frustration that a unique relationship establishes itself between a general practitioner and those of his patients who stay with him. It is very difficult to describe this relationship in psychological terms. It is not love, or mutual respect, or mutual identification, or friendship, though elements of all these enter into it. We termed it – for want of a better term – a 'mutual investment company'. By this we mean that the general practitioner gradually acquires a very valuable capital invested in his patient, and, vice versa, the patient acquires a very valuable capital bestowed in his general practitioner.[8]

Holding would seem to be different from the mutual investment company. Balint here is describing continuity of care, rather than a specifically holding relationship, although a holding relationship might be a type of unique relationship in which both GP and patient gradually 'acquire a very valuable capital'. More recently, Mechanic and Meyer explored patients' concepts of trust, and obtained a range of responses to the question, 'What does trust mean to you?':

> Trust means knowing that there's confidence in a person. That I know they'll do the right thing that's in my best interests. That the person's well trained. That they've had previous experience working on this particular type of medical problem. And that they're up to date on the latest technology, latest research. And that they treat you as an individual, as opposed to just another patient ...

Trust ... I think it's something that comes over a period of time. Trust means essentially you would trust a person with your well-being ... and in the absence of being able to control the situation, you would trust this person to control it in your best interests as well as they could.

Trust ... means compassion; it means listening and really hearing, it's just dedication. It's knowing what you tell a person is going to stay with that person.[5]

It seems inevitable that trust and holding work are intimately linked as they require much the same conditions for their development. The conditions for trust are noted above, and include confidence (which develops over a period of time) in a well-trained person who treats people as individuals, listens to them and stays with them. The conditions for holding are named in the data as constancy, being there over a period of time and on a regular basis, a longer and perhaps a deeper GP–patient relationship than usual, acceptance and valuing of the patient by the GP, support and concern, and giving time. A holding relationship implies and requires trust but is more than simply a trusting relationship.

Holding and attachment

Holding relationships have been identified in the literature of psychotherapy and offer parallels to holding in general practice. Bowlby's attachment theory (*see* reference 9 for Bowlby's own summary of this theory) offers an insight into why some patients may find it necessary to be held by their GP (or anyone else). This theory is grounded in the observation that human behaviour, from infancy onwards, includes a set of attachment behaviours which account for much of the interaction between infants and their caregivers. These behaviours are usually directed to a small number of others, they endure over a long period of time, and their alteration in any way (stopping, starting, maintaining, renewing) is associated with intense emotion. The attachment figure is seen as providing a 'secure base' under optimal conditions, allowing the infant to explore, grow progressively independent, and then show less overt attachment behaviour. Since this theory was developed based on infancy, Bowlby and others have extrapolated it to adult attachment styles.[10] In providing a holding relationship for a patient, the GP may be acting as an attachment figure, offering a 'secure base'. This may enable the patient to move on, possibly becoming progressively more independent of their need for healthcare.

Similarly, Winnicott (a child psychiatrist) described holding relationships in two ways. First, in the mother–infant relationship, holding is about both 'the physical holding of the infant which is a form of loving' and 'total environmental provision' before the emergence of the infant as a separate individual.[11] 'The mother holds a situation so that the infant has the chance to work through instinctual experiences'[12] (for a further discussion, *see* reference 13).

Second, Winnicott recognises that ego support continues to be a need of the growing child, the adolescent and, at times, the adult, whenever there is a strain which threatens confusion or disintegration. For example:

> A child is playing in the garden. An aeroplane flies low overhead. This can be hurtful even to an adult. No explanation is valuable for the child. What is valuable is that you hold the child close to yourself, and the child uses the fact that you are not scared beyond recovery, and is soon off and away, playing again.[14]

Winnicott's more metaphorical use of the concept of holding in individuals past infancy would appear to have parallels with holding work in primary care. In interim holding or episodic long-term holding, the GP holds the patient through an episode and once this has passed, the patient is free to return to his or her usual existence ('off and away, playing again'). Winnicott's holding involves being there when needed, however briefly, to facilitate maturation and integration.

However, Winnicott's holding also involves accepting an individual's current level of maturation and supporting them in this, 'counteracting disintegration',[15] even when further integration appears unlikely. The latter view of holding would fit more with continuous long-term holding, when the relationship is a 'keeping ticking over' (Paul). The individual may have a relatively constant level of maturity that requires a long-term holding relationship from the GP. The likelihood of further maturation and integration is low, and hence a long-term, more infantile, attachment is necessary.

The theories of Bowlby and Winnicott are essentially developmental, they are about moving on, maturing, developing. Holding in the general practice situation may be about this, offering the 'secure base' of the GP. But holding in general practice is equally about long-term relationships, being there, trust and constancy. These factors may be part of developing, but they may also be about support for coping and simply 'getting through'. In other words, a holding relationship in general practice can be about, first, simply being alongside, supporting or enabling an individual to maintain his or her current level of maturation ('ticking over'). Second, a holding relationship can be about allowing someone to work through issues and move on developmentally. Either of these may be a significant achievement for that individual.

Holding and problematic GP–patient relationships

A holding relationship may be useful with both frequently attending patients and heartsink patients. The reasons for establishing and managing a holding relationship are minor mental illness and subjective pathology such as loss, bereavement and relationship difficulties. Chronic physical illness is seen as needing monitoring, not holding, and more serious organic pathology is thought to require 'key worker' co-ordinating by the GP. These doctors perceive a real need in the small group of holding patients to 'come and unload', 'to sit and talk about nothing in particular,' to 'have their 10 minutes'. This relationship is generally not about cure, but about keeping people going and being there for them, in much the same way as the 'holding strategy' has been described as an approach for managing heartsink patients:

> The 'holding strategy' whereby positive attempts to bring about change are abandoned in favour of simply listening to the patient ... The doctor acts as a safety valve in the hope that changes will occur for other reasons at some time in the future. This defies medical inclinations to intervene actively ...[16]

Similarly, holding may be used to manage frequently attending patients, as some patients described as being in a holding relationship with their GP are also seen as frequent attenders, although many are not. Frequent attenders have been defined as the most frequently attending 3% of patients in general practice (corresponding to an average of at least one consultation per month).[17]

> There is one class of patient above all which contradicts the logical assumption concerning symptom cure: ... persistent attenders. ... With extraordinary persistence, they return again and again to the doctor from whom they have derived so little benefit in previous consultations. The doctor who thinks in terms of symptom removal finds these patients perplexing, frustrating and irritating.[18]

Browne and Freeling give an example, which would seem to be a holding relationship, of a frequently attending man with whom the GP:

> ... no longer tries any active therapy: both he and the patient know where they stand on this routine. ... If a doctor's work is to be thought of solely in terms of symptom cure, this consultation is simply not medicine.[18]

Developing intervention strategies around control of the pattern of consulting with frequently attending patients may be useful,[19] and designating a relationship as needing holding work is a possible strategy. Such a holding strategy may involve the GP in identifying, and negotiating with, suitable patients by naming, establishing and managing (and then understanding, accepting and reconceptualising) a maintenance (not symptom-curing) relationship.

Holding and patient-centredness

Patient-centred medicine gives priority to the personal relationship between doctor and patient:

> [The] effects of medical treatment are theoretically distinguishable from relationship effects: the former are 'real' while the latter a mysterious but potentially beneficial side-effect. In patient-centred care, however, developing a therapeutic alliance is a fundamental requirement rather than a useful addition. ... the alliance has potential therapeutic benefit in and of itself.[20]

Holding is such an alliance and may have therapeutic benefit of itself. The perceived benefit of holding work in primary care is, first, in keeping someone going or ticking over, supporting them using a GP–patient relationship that enables them to cope. Second, giving someone regular space in holding work may allow them to grow. As I have discussed, this links to psychotherapeutic theory in which holding involves accepting an individual's current level of maturation and supporting them in this, counteracting disintegration even when further integration appears unlikely.[15] It also links to psychotherapeutic theory, in which offering someone a 'secure base' allows them to gradually show less attachment behaviour and move on.[9] Such enabling relationships also link to definitions of quality in primary care. For example, Howie *et al.* suggest that:

- care delivered should improve health or halt its deterioration
- care delivered should increase the patient's ability to cope with the problem
- needs may be identified and met over a series of interactions (which may occur over a long time).[21]

The specific difference between holding work and this definition of good quality of care is that the former enables patients to cope by seeing them regularly, offering a relationship that may simply be about *maintenance* of function, without a presumption of *improvement* in function. Needs may not be met, ability to cope may not increase, but the patient is enabled to 'keep ticking over' (Paul). In everyday general practice, this is perceived as a therapeutic benefit.

Various factors influence the GP when deciding whether or not to establish a holding relationship with a particular patient, concerning either the patient or the doctor. Some doctors are firm about their boundaries and their control of the relationship, others leave it with the patient. Some find it hard to approach certain patients (such as people who are demanding). Whichever route is chosen, the person-centred dimensions of the 'patient-as-person' (the patient's needs, preferences and ideas) and the 'doctor-as-person' (the doctor's insight, self-awareness and personal boundaries) will be influential.[20] In the third and final section of this book, I consider the limits doctors establish in response to their work and discuss the doctor's self or the doctor-as-person.

References

1   Sykes J (1976) *Concise Oxford Dictionary*. Oxford University Press, Oxford.

2   Stewart-Brown S (1998) Emotional wellbeing and its relation to health. *BMJ*. **317**: 1608–9.

3   Stansfield S, Fuhrer R, Shipley M (1998) Types of support as predictors of psychiatric morbidity in a cohort of British Civil Servants (Whitehall II study). *Psychol Med*. **28**: 881–92.

4   Mookadam F, Arthur H (2004) Social support and its relationship to morbidity and mortality after acute myocardial infarction: systematic overview. *Arch Intern Med*. **164**: 1514–18.

5   Mechanic D, Meyer S (2000) Concepts of trust among patients with serious illness. *Soc Sci Med*. **51**: 657–68.

6   General Medical Council (2001) *Good Medical Practice*. General Medical Council, London.

7   Jeffs S (1973) Being a good doctor. *J R Coll Gen Pract*. **23**: 683–90.

8   Balint M (1963) *The Doctor, His Patient and the Illness* (2e). Churchill Livingstone, London.

9   Bowlby J (1977) The making and breaking of affectional bonds. *Br J Psych*. **130**: 201–10, 421–31.

10 Mace C, Margison F (1997) Attachment and psychotherapy: an overview. *Br J Med Psychol*. **70**: 209–15.

11 Winnicott D (1960) The theory of the parent–infant relationship. In: Winnicott D (1976) *The Maturational Processes and the Facilitating Environment.* The Hogarth Press, London.

12 Winnicott D (1954) The depressive position in normal emotional development. In: Winnicott D (1975) *Through Paediatrics to Psycho-analysis – Collected Papers.* The Hogarth Press, London.

13 Khan M (1986) Introduction. In: Winnicott D (ed.) *Holding and Interpretation.* The Hogarth Press, London.

14 Winnicott D (1969) Stresses at pre-school age: the building up of trust. In: Davis M, Wallbridge D (1981) *Boundary and Space: an introduction to the work of D.W. Winnicott.* Brunner/Mazel, New York.

15 Winnicott D (1963) Casework and mental illness. In: Winnicott D (1976) *The Maturational Processes and the Facilitating Environment.* The Hogarth Press, London.

16 Butler C and Evans M (1999) The 'heartsink' patient revisited. *Br J Gen Pract.* **49**: 230–3.

17 Neal R, Heywood P, Morley S *et al.* (1998) Frequency of patients' consulting in general practice and workload generated by frequent attenders: comparisons between practices. *Br J Gen Pract.* **48**: 895–8.

18 Browne K, Freeling P (1967) *The Doctor–Patient Relationship.* Livingstone, London.

19 Neal R, Heywood P, Morley S (2000) 'I always seem to be there' – a qualitative study of frequent attenders. *Br J Gen Pract.* **50**: 716–23.

20 Mead N, Bower P (2000) Patient-centredness: a conceptual framework and review of the empirical literature. *Fam Pract.* **51**: 1087–110.

21 Howie J, Heaney D, Maxwell M (1997) *Measuring Quality in General Practice.* Occasional Paper 75. Royal College of General Practitioners, London.

Section 3

Boundaries and self in listening work

8

Listening work and organisational boundaries

In Section 1, I explored listening work in GP–patient encounters, and in Section 2, I moved on to consider relationship, the consequence of cumulative listening. The first two chapters of this final section investigate pressures on these doctors in the organisation of listening work, and boundaries they negotiate in order to manage this work, both interpersonal and personal. Chapters 10 and 11 explore outcomes or effects of listening work on the doctor's self, revealing boundaries within each doctor.

Lowering of mood in GPs has been associated with 'hassle' at work, pressure of time and domestic dissatisfaction with as many as one in two GPs showing high levels of stress,[1-3] two-fifths suffering from anxiety and one-quarter from depression.[4] Pressures on each GP are imposed in part by the organisational boundaries they create in their work, and which I explore in this chapter. These may be thought of as pressures within the consultation and structural pressures in the working day, though inevitably this distinction is not clear-cut. Pressures in the consultation are mostly concerned with finding enough time for each patient. Structural pressures are created by the nature of general practice work and involve issues such as overall workload, being on call and visiting.

Pressures within the consultation

A very frequent pressure on the GP within the consultation is the patient who produces a list of problems. This may be a list written on a piece of paper or a list of complaints that gradually emerge during the consultation. Most doctors will attempt to prioritise in this situation:

> I'll say, "Hang on, just give me your piece of paper. That's four problems all of at least one appointment each. Sorry, pick the most important one

and we'll deal with that today. Then come back and we'll deal with the others".' (Ben)

Some doctors find prioritisation a problem in itself:

'If they've come with three things, I nearly always end up touching on all of them, rather than say, "We'll leave that to another day completely".' (Paul)

This puts the doctor under pressure and may mean that issues are not covered ideally. Most difficult is:

'When people don't say they've got three problems' (Don)

and each problem is presented on completion of the previous one. This is a well-recognised situation and is much less easy to prioritise.

A useful time management tool is to identify a list of problems and then postpone dealing with some of them until a future occasion, rather than attempting to manage several issues within the time constraints of a single consultation. Some GPs have several ways of saying, 'Can you come back another time?' and this is thought to be acceptable, on the whole, to patients:

'Well we can't really talk about it now, will you come and see me this evening or tomorrow?' (Tim)

'Look, this is a complicated case, there's a lot more to do, make a double appointment tomorrow or the day after, let's come back and in the meantime I'd like you to write some notes for me and tell me.' (Chaz)

'Hang on, I know where we need to be going here but we can't do it today. We need to be fair to me and to you and to everybody else out there, let's get you back with a bit more time.' (Rick)

' "My next patient's waiting, we don't need to deal with this immediately today, here's a plan to be going on with while you're waiting to see me." I'm always amazed that you can see somebody three weeks later, and it's like we've picked up the conversation again. There is no gap, there is no catch-up time, the consultation begins where it left off.' (Ed)

Other methods of coping with these pressures, such as seeing fewer patients or offering longer or double appointments, can create additional pressures for the GP. This is because the question arises of:

'What is a valid use of time in the general practice context?' (Chris)

Within this question is the subtext of 'Who defines what is valid?'. On the one hand, having a longer consultation may make both doctor and patient more relaxed and satisfied, and create the impetus to sort out more than one problem in each consultation. On the other, giving one person more time may well mean giving another person less time or seeing fewer people in that surgery. While variation may be achieved by the natural flexibility of the surgery:

> 'It's swings and roundabouts; we do so many in an hour and if one is longer than the others, you can catch up.' (Alex)

it may also create significant workload issues for the doctor.

Seeing people for longer in a surgery may be achieved by giving the patient a double appointment or giving them the last appointment of the surgery. Several pressures may arise from giving a double appointment:

> 'The problem with blanking out two is that you are less available for all the others.' (Steve)

> 'If I use up too much of my appointment time with double appointments, then I am seeing fewer people. I would feel guilty.' (Ben)

> 'I'm not taking my fair share of the workload.' (Chris)

This guilt may be 'a mental thing' for the individual doctor, unnoticed within the partnership. Often there is an informal consensus, or occasionally a formal agreement, that double appointments should be avoided:

> 'Double appointments are frowned upon. We feel it's a way of making surgery a bit easier. ... We tend to say, "Find time elsewhere in your timetable".' (Matt)

> 'We don't book longer appointments, we're not allowed to. One partner used to do that a lot and it looked like she was seeing a lot fewer patients, so there was a lot of jealousy around. The rules are we have to stick to seven and a half minute appointments.' (Phil)

This sort of partnership arrangement restricting and limiting the format of the surgery, whether informal or more formal, puts additional pressures on doctors, particularly when patients are thought to require extra time or if the individual doctor 'does not buy into the agreement':

'I don't think you can do your job properly in seven and half minutes. It can get irritating because you do your normal workload and add on, but you have to do that in your own conscience to do your job properly. But you question, "Does everybody else do it?". This makes me sound as though I've got a gripe but that's where I think workloads can never be equal because we don't practise the same sort of medicine. It can get under your skin and I believe you should be honest and have that out in the open. I think if you let things like that rumble on, they can cause problems. You wonder if you're just being pedantic, whether other practices have the same problems. We're human beings and we have to take that into the equation. We're supposed to come in here and be a doctor with no other personal pressures. I'm getting to the point where I don't believe that that's right.' (Sam)

'When I first started in general practice, it used to be a fairly accepted thing that these people came in [for longer chats], but then I think people found themselves having to justify how they spent time with people. Whether that came from partners or it came from external influences, … they had to look critically at what time they spent with people. Maybe it's a bad thing, maybe people did more good by being more in contact with the patients.' (Ed)

Working arrangements, such as issues of workload equality and booked length of appointment, tend to be decided between the partners in a practice (who will often have different opinions and outlooks) with a variety of effects.[5,6] Some partners are keen to allow time to listen whereas others:

'… may not feel that is a valid use of time.' (Chris)

A fair share of the workload seems to mean seeing the same number of patients as everyone else, irrespective of the appointment length – a lowest common denominator approach? This is noted as a perennial difficulty in some practices.

Structural pressures in the working day

As I have already highlighted in Chapter 3, the chief pressure in the structure of the working day for these doctors is lack of time, and this is a constant awareness in their minds. How to use time most efficiently and what constitutes a valid use of time in general practice are key questions. The practical application of the answers to these questions, at a personal level and a partnership level, sets the tone for the amount of structural pressure on each GP. I have discussed some aspects of managing time and listening already in Chapter 3.

The central structure in the working day of the average GP is the surgery, composed of consultations with patients or groups of patients. The format for each surgery is generally agreed between the partners, formally or informally, so that workload is shared. The extent to which agreement can be obtained for this format, and the realities of applying it in everyday general practice work, create a great many of the structural pressures on these doctors. Agreed formats reported within a partnership involve each doctor seeing up to 15 or 20 patients in a surgery. Appointment lengths, generally of between seven and ten minutes per patient, may be fixed by each individual partner, uniform for all the doctors in the partnership or, exceptionally, specified by the patient. Such formats, balancing organisational structure with individual agency, have the advantage of providing a transparent equality to the workload between the doctors, but they are also observed to create numerous pressures.

The most common pressure is that of running late. The majority of these doctors are realistic about the fact that they 'will always run late' (Sam), although the amount of pressure this creates varies from doctor to doctor:

'It's a good surgery when I overrun by less than 30 minutes.' (Ben)

'I always run late – by and large the patients don't suffer.' (Rick)

'If you run 20 patient surgeries, booked at eight minutes but running probably at 10–12 (minutes), then it all stacks up.' (Ben)

'A few years ago I was more uptight about things like that and I used to think, "I've got to keep roughly to time in the surgery". Now I'm much more relaxed about it, my surgery finishes when it finishes. I try and do my best but I think the patients who see me know that I won't necessarily run to time, but they also know that if they've got a problem, they will have time to talk about it.' (Pete)

A few doctors report always running to time:

'I stick to my appointment times because I think it's a contract with the patient and I think you can effectively manage the consultation.' (Ed)

The computer on the doctor's desk may not help the pressure building as the surgery runs late:

'Since we've been computerised, the surgery list is on the screen, in front of you. When you're consulting, you see the times that people come and you see this little line stacking up, like in the airport when the planes can't take off. I find that creates pressure and reflects itself in how you deal with more complicated cases.' (Huw)

Outside formal surgery times, other organisation of workload comes into consideration. The list identified is extensive and includes home visits, telephone calls, paperwork, meetings, visits to residential and nursing homes, work in local hospitals, medical examinations, coil fits and family planning clinics, minor operations, visits to branch surgeries, practice administration and teaching medical students and GP registrars. Added to this is taking a share in being duty doctor for the day, when any activity may be interrupted at any time by demands and emergencies, with consequent knock-on time pressures for other activities later in the day.

If several doctors are away or there are numerous extra visits that day, then there is likely to be little time to allow 'space to expand' (Tom) within the consultation. Locum doctors can also create pressure because it is thought that they may not get fully to the bottom of some listening issues, causing the patient to return and creating extra work for the partners.

The restraints of the format of the day, and the time pressures it creates, are seen as the key structural pressures for these doctors:

'I think the only pressure is the time constraints and keeping it within a system. That's the difficult bit.' (Pete)

Several methods of coping with these pressures and organising time were discussed. Delegation of some activities, remaining relaxed when under pressure, developing skills in time management, and the ability to prioritise:

'I'd like to get involved with all that, but I don't have the time' (Matt)

are all important. Home visiting is increasingly seen as inefficient:

'If they can get to the hairdresser, they can get to the surgery.' (Matt)

Although some visits, for example to the housebound, cannot be avoided, offering a consultation at the surgery, immediately or in the near future, is seen as a better use of the GP's time.

Having enough time in the consultation is important to these doctors and this concern is also evident in the literature of primary care. When more time is made available in the consultation, better communication occurs between doctors and patients[7] and there is considerable evidence[8] showing the benefits of longer consultations (seven and a half or ten minutes against five minutes; *see* Box 8.1).

Box 8.1 Evidence favouring longer booking intervals*

- In consultations booked at five-minute, compared with ten-minute, intervals, doctors identified fewer problems and recorded blood pressure fewer times, and patients were less satisfied
- In those consultations booked at ten-minute intervals, doctors spent more time discussing clinical problems and management, and health education and prevention
- More psychosocial issues were dealt with in longer consultations and fewer antibiotics were prescribed
- Lower levels of stress in doctors are demonstrated with ten-minute booking intervals

---

* Adapted from Williams & Neal (1998)[9]

Longer consultation times allow patients to ask more questions and more fully express their own ideas.[10] They also allow more discussion of lifestyle factors, with more screening and health promotion activity.[11,12] The difficulty is actually creating adequate time in everyday practice when demand for healthcare is rising,[5,13] along with the workload of GPs.[14,15] One possibility to create adequate time would be small practices with few patients per doctor. There have been arguments for and against this option,[16–18] and the underlying assumption (that fewer patients per doctor will allow improvements in existing care) has been questioned.[19] Smaller practices report improved accessibility of care and better continuity of care compared with larger practices,[20] but defining optimal practice size is complex and influenced by other factors (for example, socio-economic deprivation[21] and the use of nurse practitioners).[22] Patients are known to prefer smaller practices,[23] but doctors can impose their own patterns of work whatever the size or composition of their list.[24]

As I have already noted, consultation rates arranged in appointment systems also influence the creation of time in everyday practice. The number of appointments per week needed to meet anticipated demand can be calculated,[25,26] allowing for variations in rates between ethnic groups[27] and age, sex and disability.[28] Flexibility within systems may be created by allowing patients to choose the length of their appointment[29–31] or by introducing 'advanced access'.[32–34] However, implementing such change in consultation bookings can be complicated,[33] though it may lead to measureable improvement in outcomes such as doctor and patient satisfaction.[35]

In the literature of general practice, and for these doctors, the common factor in organising the structure of the working day is creating time, which directly influences pressure in the consultation. Additionally, there is no doubt that workloads differ from doctor to doctor because of the way each individual interprets their role as a GP. This creates varying pressures within each person influenced by external pressures from partners and patients alike. In the next chapter, I discuss some of these interpersonal factors.

References

1   Caplan R (1994) Stress, anxiety and depression in hospital consultants, general practitioners and senior health service managers. *BMJ.* **309**: 1261–3.

2   Appleton K, House A, Dowell A (1998) A survey of job satisfaction, sources of stress and psychological symptoms among general practitioners in Leeds. *Br J Gen Pract.* **48**: 1059–63.

3   Dowell A, Hamilton S, Mcleod D (2000) Job satisfaction, psychological morbidity and job stress among New Zealand general practitioners. *N Z Med J.* **113**: 269–72.

4   Chambers R, Campbell I (1996) Anxiety and depression in general practitioners: associations with type of practice, fund-holding, gender and other personal characteristics. *Fam Pract.* **13**: 170–3.

5   Huby G, Gerry M, McKinstry B *et al.* (2002) Morale among general practitioners: qualitative study exploring relations between partnership arrangements, personal style and workload. *BMJ.* **325**: 140–2.

6   Branson R, Armstrong D (2004) General practitioners' perceptions of sharing workload in group practices: qualitative study. *BMJ.* **329**: 381–4.

7   Roland M, Bartholomew J, Courtenay MJF *et al.* (1986) The 'five minute' consultation: effect of time constraint on verbal communication. *BMJ.* **292**: 874–6.

8   Wilson A, Childs S (2002) The relationship between consultation length, process and outcomes in general practice: a systematic review. *Br J Gen Pract.* **52**: 1012–20.

9   Williams M, Neal R (1998) Time for a change? The process of lengthening booking intervals in general practice. *Br J Gen Pract.* **48**: 1783–6.

10 Ridsdale L, Carruthers M, Morris R *et al.* (1989) Study of the effect of time availability on the consultation. *J Roy Coll Gen Pract.* **39**: 488–91.

11 Wilson A (1989) Extending appointment length – the effect in one practice. *J Roy Coll Gen Pract.* **39**: 24–5.

12   Wilson A, McDonald P, Hayes L *et al.* (1992) Health promotion in the general practice consultation: a minute makes a difference. *BMJ.* **304**: 227–30.

13   Pencheon D (1998) Matching demand and supply fairly and efficiently. *BMJ.* **316**: 1665–7.

14   Chambers R, Belcher J (1993) Work patterns of general practitioners before and after the introduction of the 1990 contract. *Br J Gen Pract.* **43**: 410–12.

15   Kavanagh S, Knapp M (1998) The impact on general practitioners of the changing balance of care for elderly people living in institutions. *BMJ.* **317**: 322–7.

16   Marsh G (1991) Caring for larger lists. *BMJ.* **303**: 1312–16.

17   Knight R (1987) The importance of list size and consultation length as factors in general practice. *J Roy Coll Gen Pract.* **37**: 19–22.

18   Campbell J (1996) The reported availability of general practitioners and the influence of practice list size. *Br J Gen Pract.* **46**: 465–8.

19   Butler J, Calnan M (1987) List sizes and use of time in general practice. *BMJ.* **295**: 1383–6.

20   Campbell J, Ramsey J, Green J (2001) Practice list size: impact on consultation length, workload, and patient assessment of care. *Br J Gen Pract.* **51**: 644–50.

21   Stirling A, Wilson P, McConnachie A (2001) Deprivation, psychological distress, and consultation length in general practice. *Br J Gen Pract.* **51**: 456–60.

22   Laurant M, Hermens R, Braspenning J *et al.* (2004) Impact of nurse practitioners on workload of general practitioners: randomised controlled trial. *BMJ.* **328**: 927–30.

23   Baker R, Streatfield J (1995) What type of general practice do patients prefer? Exploration of practice characteristics influencing patient satisfaction. *Br J Gen Pract.* **45**: 654–9.

24   Day P, Klein R (1987) General practice: a blurred snapshot. *BMJ.* **295**: 253–5.

25   Fleming D (1989) Consultation rates in English general practice. *J Roy Coll Gen Pract.* **39**: 68–72.

26   Campbell J, Howie J (1992) Changes resulting from increasing appointment length: practical and theoretical issues. *Br J Gen Pract.* **42**: 276–8.

27   Gillam S, Jarman B, White P *et al.* (1989) Ethnic differences in consultation rates in urban general practice. *BMJ.* **299**: 533–7.

28   Hall R, Channing D (1990) Age, pattern of consultation, and functional disability in elderly patients in one general practice. *BMJ.* **301**: 424–8.

29   Lowenthal L, Bingham E (1987) Length of consultation: how well do patients choose? *J Roy Coll Gen Pract.* **37**: 498–9.

30   Harrison A (1988) Appointment systems: evaluation of a flexible system offering patients limited choice. *BMJ.* **296**: 685–6.

31   Pascoe S, Neal R, Allgar V (2004) Open-access versus bookable appointment systems: survey of patients attending appointments with general practitioners. *Br J Gen Pract.* **54**: 367–9.

32   Oldham J (2001) *Advanced Access in Primary Care.* National Primary Care Development Team, Manchester.

33   Murray M, Bodenheimer T, Rittenhouse D, Grumbach K (2003) Improving timely access to primary care: case studies of the advanced access model. *JAMA.* **289**: 1042–6.

34   Pickin M, Cathain C, Sampson F *et al.* (2004) Evaluation of advanced access in the primary care collaborative. *Br J Gen Pract.* **54**: 334–40.

35   Williams M, Neal R (1998) Time for a change? The process of lengthening booking intervals in general practice. *Br J Gen Pract.* **48**: 1783–6.

9

Listening work and interpersonal boundaries

Interpersonal pressures for the GP arise in a variety of ways. Those occurring between doctors in the allocation and structuring of the daily schedule and workload have been described in the previous chapter. Those occurring between doctors and their patients are equally complex. Central to these pressures is the interpersonal distance or boundary between GP and patient.

Some doctors express considerable feelings of attachment towards their patients, whereas others try to remain more distant:

'I was too nice I think. I liked him too much to be tough with him. I felt he needed someone who could be very tough with him.' (Chris)

'It would be impossible to do the job and enjoy it without having feelings and sometimes those feelings are very deep about some individuals. It hurts when I've had to work very hard to resolve problems and they get up and walk out of the room.' (Tom)

'I think we are supposed to counsel the patient and give advice and comment. We should divorce ourselves from what actually we feel ourselves.' (Chaz)

Such separating of the professional self from the personal self can be a struggle:

'When she was first diagnosed, I was very upset. Every time she came in, she'd burst into floods of tears and it was a struggle for me not to burst into floods of tears with her. One day I did a little bit, but I was trying all the time to reassure her and it was quite hard at times because I was upset about it myself and trying to distance myself and just all the time give her positive vibes. Emotionally I was very involved and I did have to try and step back and deal with it in my own time.' (Vic)

The pressures and anxieties of these emotional attachments are increased by a pre-existing relationship of some kind, narrowing the interpersonal distance between GP and patient. This might be knowing the patient's family, knowing the patient as a friend or a colleague (particularly a fellow doctor or other health professional), meeting the patient through other activities or at school, or even employing the patient either at the surgery or in the doctor's home. Significant events happening to people with whom the GP identifies, such as people of the same age and sex as either the GP or a member of the doctor's family, also narrow the interpersonal distance between doctor and patient:

'I had three men all in their mid-fifties who died in the space of two months. It makes you look at your mortality. I'm that age. It's getting a bit close to home when it happens like that and you see the impact of those deaths on families that expected to be a family unit for a lot longer. It does make you look at things and realise what's important to you.' (Huw)

'The only time when I found it upsetting was when a little girl was dying exactly the same age as my daughter. There was a part of me that was grieving through all that. There's a warm professional part to do and you feel that everything is going well. There's another side that's the bit grieving alongside that's got to be completely blocked off and in control and capable of being independent. Boxed off, in control and doing the professional bit.' (Tom)

As has been noted, interpersonal pressures arise from alterations in the interpersonal and emotional distance or boundary between GP and patient. The remainder of this chapter considers situations in which the GP–patient encounter may become more 'personal' and less 'professional', the interpersonal distance may narrow with shifting of boundaries, and the doctor's degree of emotional involvement with the patient may alter.

Friendliness and GP–patient relationships

Discussion of boundaries between patients as patients and patients as friends divides into four sub-sections. In the first group are 'people who are very much patients and that's how it always is', with fairly clear boundaries. There may be many of these patients who are 'almost friends', but in the context of the clear statement that 'one would like to think that 90% of our patients are friends'. In other words, this level of friendship is to do with friendliness and mutual respect within a routine doctor–patient interaction:

> 'I think friends is a difficult term because there are different types of friends aren't there? I think there's a difference between friends and friendly in a way. There are patients with whom I am more friendly than others. The longer you're here, you see people more and more frequently, and so I suppose the more you see them, the more a friendship arises, but that friendship is only about their medical problems. In the context of a surgery, if you feel a friendship towards a patient, I think that's fine.' (Will)

In this situation, it is reasonably easy to be clear that friendliness is a product of the long-term professional relationship, and neither the doctor nor the patient wishes to change the balance of the relationship.

Patients who want to be friends

The second group contains 'patients who want to be more friendly' with their GP. Within this group boundaries are less clear and dilemmas for the GP arise. The following excerpt illustrates some of the issues.

> SC   'I had this chap who took me climbing once, but it felt a bit odd. It felt like he wanted to move from just an ordinary patient doctor– relationship.'
>
> Lee   'So you weren't friends before?'
>
> SC   'No, no. And he was trying to alter it. It felt a bit odd and it was quite obvious that it wasn't going to be a social thing. It was going to stay as an ordinary doctor–patient relationship but he wanted to be more than just an ordinary patient.'
>
> Lee   'I don't encourage that, to be honest. I do prefer it to be a professional relationship between doctor and patient and I think it does change your relationship if that does happen. I've got a patient who always buys me gifts and I don't like it, but I don't know how to say "no". I almost feel as if it's a sort of bribe in a way. It's a funny feeling, and they're always very nice gifts and quite expensive gifts. Christmas, all sorts of occasions, any excuse to bring a parcel in, and

> I don't feel comfortable with that because when you see that patient
> again, you think, "This patient's given me gifts". I don't want to alter
> my doctor relationship in any way compared with any of my other
> patients just because this particular patient brings me gifts. It feels
> odd and I suppose the next thing on from that is developing a
> friendship with somebody and then trying to alter that relationship
> which does feel uncomfortable really. Trying to establish a friendship
> within the doctor–patient relationship would feel strange and would
> feel uncomfortable. GPs who live in the local area do have friends
> who they see as patients. But it's the other way round, they're
> friends initially.'

An invitation from a patient to go fishing, walking, or whatever, will
generally feel:

> '… almost a bridge too far. We are closer than average but at the end of
> the day, I don't want to get too close. But now we are talking about
> situations where really they still are patients and all your contact with
> them, albeit wider than the average consultation, is through the consulta-
> tion, and they are wanting to take it a step further, and that I am not
> comfortable with.' (Rick)

With some patients a gradual alteration in the interpersonal distance over
time is described and relates, for example, to the closeness often resulting
from managing a chronic or life-threatening illness. Respondents would
consider it appropriate for the boundaries of this relationship to change in the
direction of increased friendliness, but not towards friendship:

> 'The more you see them, the more a friendship arises but that friendship is
> only about their medical problems and that's OK in the context of a
> surgery. I don't think, as a result of that type of friendship, I have ever said,
> "Shall we go and have a game of golf?" or "Should we do that?". What I've
> relied on is when I play golf, I meet another set of people with whom I
> may become friendly because of the golf. I think I'm pretty careful at
> drawing that line.' (Will)

These patients are seen quite clearly by their GPs to have an appropriate
doctor–patient relationship, which is valued but which equally remains
friendliness in the context of a professional relationship, as distinct from *friendship*. Attempting to establish a friendship on the basis of the doctor–patient
relationship in the surgery is uncomfortable and rarely satisfactory. Only
one exception to this was described in which the GP has developed a

long-standing and firm friendship, away from the medical relationship, with a patient who suffers from recurrent illness.

Some patients are thought to be seeking, either consciously or unconsciously, to create a fundamental change in the relationship, perhaps from friendliness to friendship. Although some doctors welcome and encourage use of their first name by all their patients, for others this is, if uninvited, an uncomfortable closing of distance between doctor and patient. The patient who constantly buys their GP presents, or who offers repeated invitations to social events, may leave the GP feeling bribed and uncomfortable in the implications that this has for the doctor–patient relationship. Reciprocal favours can be expected and there is the fear of being manipulated for preferential treatment.

Patients who bring presents to their GP highlight decisions on where to limit the GP–patient relationship. Such presents and their givers seem to fall into three categories: those that feel comfortable and appropriate to the GP; those that feel uncomfortable but not inappropriate; and those that feel both uncomfortable and inappropriate. The former include the:

> '... little old lady who brings a pot of jam and likes a social chat about the doctor's children' (Lew)

along with her own medical care, and the occasional cards and bottles at Christmas time or after a particular episode of illness. Those that feel uncomfortable but not inappropriate are the friendly patients who always give a Christmas present or bring alcohol, who are thought to expect a little extra time and a warmer relationship. The last category, uncomfortable and inappropriate, includes people whom these doctors find difficult or awkward. In these situations, the gifts, which are sometimes frequent and invariably unwanted, are perceived as a bribe which may put pressure on the GP. Gifts from patients to their GP, and the reaction elicited, perhaps both symbolise and reflect the nature of the relationship of that patient with that GP.

Friends as patients

The third group is 'people who are friends and also patients'. This group is 'friends who really are friends'. Boundary and distance seem clear, particularly with people who have been personal friends away from the surgery for some time:

> 'I feel comfortable with patients who are friends when they have started as friends almost before you discovered they were patients, or the friendship

is developed away from being a patient. It's been two separate things. I've got quite a few people, even really close friends, who are patients and I'm comfortable with that completely.' (Paul)

A few of the doctors interviewed:

'... haven't got any friends who are patients because I don't think you can mix the two. They tend to abuse their privileged position of knowing your phone number and ringing you when you're not on duty. That really annoys me, I'm very aware of my own protected time. A very large brick wall between surgery and home.' (Alex)

Generally, 'friends who are also patients' work hard to respect boundaries between friendship and being a patient:

'Friend friends wouldn't put you in an awkward situation I don't think. If it's their decision, they wouldn't want to talk about anything medical when you're on a friend basis and if they come to the surgery, it's almost very formal. They would just like to be like anyone else. But the people who have decided that you're going to be their friend will have no hesitation in bumping their trolley into yours and saying, "Oh, by the way, those tablets you gave me last week. ...".' (Tim)

The contrast is clear. Similarly, it is perceived that true 'friend friends' will always ring the doctor on call if the situation arises, rather than contacting their friend who happens to be their GP as well.

These doctors have some concerns about friends who also happen to be patients. First, they tend to be overcautious, feeling under pressure to investigate, refer or prescribe when normally reassurance would suffice. It is a worry that 'having friends as patients can cloud your clinical judgement' and there is a tendency 'to try harder'. Second, there are concerns about confidentiality and remembering what has been said at the surgery that should not be repeated elsewhere. Third, psychological or relationship problems and major or life-threatening illness in this group can create enormous pressures for the GP. For example, marital difficulties may result in the GP being 'the friend at night and the doctor during the day'. A small group of doctors were adamant that they would 'never again' take a friend from diagnosis to death or through a marriage breakdown – 'once bitten, twice shy' was the feeling. Lastly, treating the children or family of friends creates the same concerns.

In addition to illness in friends who are patients, concerns and boundary issues arise when friends who are patients of other GPs develop an illness:

'I got him down to the physiotherapist. In my view, he was being less than adequately treated so I stepped in, and I would do that. I manage to stay aside most of the time and I try not to get involved. I wouldn't, as a friend, go round and put any pressure on the doctor or deliberately try and influence management unless I felt it was wrong. If it was wrong, I would tell them. I wouldn't just stand by and say nothing.' (Pete)

Involvement in the management of a friend by a colleague creates dilemmas, particularly when there is unhappiness with that management or the two doctors do not get on with each other.

Doctors as patients

Having other doctors as patients presents unique challenges and puts particular pressures on the GP, but many issues that arise are the same as those for patients as friends. The most commonly mentioned difficulty:

'... is getting the middle line. Either you give too much reassurance and say "forget it" or you go completely the other way and do too many investigations and referrals, maybe even have things done that do not need to be done.' (Vic)

There is a tendency to be over-cautious, to be afraid of making mistakes and generally attempt to bend over backwards for colleagues and staff to obtain the most appropriate treatment. Doctors do not get the same consultations as other patients because:

'It is impossible to forget that they are a doctor and treat them like anybody else.' (Vic)

It can be difficult to say:

'You've got to be ill here. Let's get you right. I'm your doctor.' (Rick)

The same GP is quite clear about these boundaries:

'I don't think I've had any problems along those regards and I do have colleagues as patients or people in the profession, who've come to see me. We actually have to address that as a potential problem often right at the start, because I think far too often we suffer by somebody trying to treat us differently to the way we would treat another patient. I think most people would say, "Just treat me as you would anybody else" because it works out better that way. Obviously you do make allowances, you will have a quiet word with the consultant and say, "This is so and so who is a GP". There aren't many perks working in the health service, and I think for anybody that's working in it, whether it be a doctor or whether it be a nurse or even just a porter or something like that, to get a bit of prefer-ential treatment is not asking a lot. I would *do* the same things.' (Rick)

Additionally, extra pressure may be created if a doctor has a problem that is psychological or psychiatric rather than physical. It may be hard for the doctor as patient to acknowledge and possibly difficult for the doctor as physician to confront.

Also described is difficulty maintaining the doctor–patient relationship with ex-colleagues or with colleagues' spouses. This can feel too close and the level of trust can feel 'overwhelming'. Examples included treating a revered ex-colleague, taking an ex-colleague through a terminal illness or relating to an ex-colleague who still expects to be treated as a colleague and co-worker. Lack of confidence, anxiety, fear of failure and a feeling of being under pressure are described in working with this group as patients. It is difficult to establish suitable boundaries and remain neutral:

'Treating colleagues is fraught with difficulty. It's probably better to go to somebody you've never met before in your life.' (Matt)

Place and interpersonal boundaries

Patients whom the GP 'knows roughly, semi-acquaintances', already known in some way or another outside the doctor–patient relationship, may assume, correctly or incorrectly, that their relationship with the GP is somehow different. Neighbours are noted sometimes to call the GP at home rather than contacting the surgery or expect the doctor–patient relationship, and hence often the consultation, to extend into the street or the back garden. This may be quite acceptable to the doctor, or may create awkwardness and interfere with the normal neighbour–neighbour relationship. Acquaintances known, for example, through sporting contact, through shared children's activities or through the doctor's spouse are all reported sometimes to have expectations which create pressure for the GP.

Other pressures occur, and interpersonal limits alter, when the GP is approached away from the surgery. Venues mentioned include the school playground, the supermarket, the waiting room of the cottage hospital, at local sporting events and in the street. Reasons given include passport forms, test results, anxiety, shotgun certificates and general advice. Approaches away from the surgery create worries for doctors, particularly about confidentiality, not listening properly, remembering what has been said or done, making mistakes, knowing what level to take people at, feeling embarrassed about the clinical topic being discussed (such as a gynaecological issue) and taking on colleagues' responsibilities. Strategies for dealing with these approaches include feeling happy and rewarded by talking to patients in the street, being only prepared to talk generally (but not specifically) away from the surgery, and having a clear boundary that the surgery is the correct and only place for such interactions ('you need a few little putdowns for the aisles at Sainsbury's').

In this chapter, we have seen that some patients are thought to want to change the balance of their relationship with their GP, from friendliness to friendship. Fears, from the doctor's perspective, of crossing the friend–patient boundary have been expressed for many years:

> It is hard to get a good history from the patient known well socially. One does not like delving into his life to the extent which is required in history taking. He will resent questions as being too personal, though before coming to the surgery, he may have intended telling everything.[1]

> Treating relatives and friends: look before you leap![2]

I have explored judgements by doctors about interpersonal distance between doctor and patient by focusing on friendliness and friendship in the doctor–patient encounter. Mostly, the judgement is straightforward: either interpersonal distance is not an issue ('patients who are always patients') or an acceptable position is easily established ('friends who are patients'). On the whole, this latter group ('friend friends') appear to respect the boundaries of their GP friends, though judging appropriate involvement in major problems (such as marital issues or terminal illness) appears to be a boundary that is learnt by experience.

However, there is a small group of patients ('patients who wish to be friends') who are seen to need, for whatever reason, to push on the boundary and attempt to vary the interpersonal distance. Patients have been reported to transgress the limit of the doctor–patient relationship[3] and actively to test the doctor's personal or professional boundary.[4] Attempts to vary interpersonal distance by patients, such as symbolically with presents or in situations away from the surgery, can leave doctors feeling uncomfortable, embarrassed or awkward. Such behaviour has been described as a 'manipulative' attempt to change distance in the nurse–patient relationship.[5] It is clear that it is exceptional for a patient to establish friendship and become a true 'friend

friend' – almost invariably, any variation in distance, or change in relationship, remains limited to friendliness within the context of a professional doctor–patient relationship.

The examples discussed in this section create dilemmas, which vary for each GP, in knowing where to position interpersonal boundaries and where to draw the line for each patient or group of patients. Judgements concerning interpersonal distance or limits in doctor–patient relationships are made subject, first, to situational factors (structure), such as the organisational pressures reported in Chapter 8, particularly time (availability, management, and arrangements within practices). Second, they are influenced by the individuals involved (agency). A variety of factors and responses in the doctor's self have been identified in this chapter, which subjectively affect interpersonal distance between patient and doctor. I explore these further in the next two chapters.

References

1   Shorten O (1966) The doctor–patient relationship in the surgery. *J Coll Gen Pract.* **11**: 21–7.

2   Bonke B, Bouman C (2000) Treating relatives and friends: look before you leap! *Br J Gen Pract.* **50**: 428–9.

3   Farber N, Novack D, O'Brien M (1997) Love, boundaries and the patient–physician relationship. *Arch Intern Med.* **157**: 2291–4.

4   Gore J, Ogden J (1998) Developing, validating and consolidating the doctor–patient relationship: patients' views of a dynamic process. *Br J Gen Pract.* **48**: 1391–4.

5   Morse J (1991) Negotiating commitment and involvement in the nurse–patient relationship. *J Adv Nurs.* **16**: 455–68.

10

Work and self: boundaries

In this chapter, I investigate the limits or personal boundaries doctors impose on the overlap between their personal and home life and their work. The effects of such strategies on doctors are explored, revealing something of the doctor's self or person (previously little described in the literature of patient-centred medicine[1]) with consequent interior or subjective boundaries.

Work, home and boundaries

When attempting to disentangle home and work, boundaries on availability are created. There is a strong consensus that it is important to stick to the working day, and not to feel guilty about finishing a full day's work at 6pm or thereabouts when tiredness is creeping in. It is emphasised, in the context of being a caring GP, both that:

> 'The days of going home at 8pm have gone (because you don't go home for a three-hour lunch break)' (Sam)

and that it is legitimate to have home, family and other commitments:

> 'I've got a life.' (Sam)

> 'Work is work and the rest isn't.' (Jo)

> 'By the time I've finished, I'm pretty shattered, so I'm ready to come home. Home life is important. Medicine is a means to earn your money to enjoy life and you've got to draw the line somewhere. So I try and get home, and I try not to bring work home. I try and switch off.' (Pete)

Some doctors aim never to bring work home. They either stay longer at the surgery or come back in the evening or at the weekend.

The boundary between home and work is brought clearly into focus by the doctor's decision on where to live, in or out of the practice area. Some doctors feel committed to being available locally, whereas others are happy to live further away:

'I'm the only doctor in the practice who's actually not ex-directory. I never really felt that we should go ex-directory. I might do in time because I'm getting more calls, but I've felt that if there is something urgent, we should be available whatever happened. That's why I live in the town as well. You've got to be somewhat available. Old-fashioned really.' (Pete)

'I actually do genuinely relish not being there because I really think it would intrude. I still think about the patients but there is a certain protection of not being right there. If I lived right next door, I could see myself popping round and running errands for people which I think is beyond the boundaries really.' (Chris)

Another doctor described moving to live out of the practice area as:

'. . . a big help because I can wander round and nobody knows who I am. But if I wander around in the practice patch, all sorts of people say "Hello" and even come for consultations in the shops.' (Steve)

Interruptions and demands when not on duty are seen by a small minority of doctors as part of living among their patients in a semi-rural community:

'I wasn't on call, but you feel obliged to go. It's difficult. I went out and sorted it out. It happens quite frequently and I just take it as part and parcel of being a GP in an area like this and being here for a long time and knowing a lot of people and I don't mind it. It is a bit of an imposition. I don't think you'd get the same if you were downtown.' (Chaz)

Most of these GPs are very clear about their boundaries of availability when off duty:

'Some colleagues in the past were quite happy for patients to have their private number and perhaps ring them at any time, but we don't have that. Certainly people can contact us any time during the day, but at six o'clock the phone goes over and I wouldn't expect somebody to contact me at night.' (Tim)

Persistent problems with a few patients who do not respect this boundary were described. One doctor:

'... had to be blunt before he [the patient] got the message that I was off-duty.' (Alex)

Practical boundaries may have to be introduced, such as a change of home telephone number or a machine that:

'... tells me the number of the person who is phoning in order to stop people who do not respect the fact that I have time to myself.' (Alex)

The exceptions reported to everything that has been said so far about availability in this section are terminal care and bereavement. In these key areas, boundaries are different. When seeing patients and their families in such situations, these doctors regularly make sure that they have extra time, that they are not under pressure and that they are able to give as much as required:

'... because you've just got one chance.' (Jo)

'I don't think that I've got limits in the terminal care or bereavement situation, or if I have, I haven't found them. They'll have my home number, I'll go in on my way home or before I go to bed or whatever. It's an area of care which I find rewarding.' (Tom)

Availability is also influenced by another boundary – doctors' perceptions of their relationship or degree of involvement with a patient:

'Ones you respect, you tend to become a little more friendly with. You tend to give them that extra bit of time or advice or lay yourself open a little bit more availability-wise. They tend to be characters that you get on with so that they aren't stressful for you. The ones that are stressful, you tend to keep at arm's length or put a block on.' (Sam)

As I discussed in Chapter 4, at any one time some patients are particularly significant for their GP:

'He's special, I saved his life.' (Matt)

An example would be a patient who is:

'... a pleasant person to talk to and a smiley face, even with serious illness. Yes, I was quite upset when he suddenly died. I have a feeling that I'm missing him, that somebody who was quite cheerful and funny isn't going to be there any more. There's a feeling of something gone. He was a friendly chap, and a nice bloke to meet and you miss that.' (Ben)

Some GPs feel able to detach themselves from their patients and their illnesses. Others worry about, for example, the threat of inappropriate emotional attachments noted in Chapter 3, or about patients who are dependent or demanding. Some think about patients away from work and may lie awake at night worrying about them. Separating work and home can be difficult:

'You have to disentangle the garbage that's running around your brain. Monday morning, you've had a weekend away, not particularly wanting to be back at work, trying to get all the red wine you had on Saturday night out of the system. So there's lots of garbage and I think you've got to remain alert. I may behave one way on one day in one set of circumstances and the patient may get a different reaction another day depending on what the pressures are. I try to keep those external pressures away so I can see each person as a different encounter. But things like, "I've got to ring the bank" – you can't always keep those things out completely.' (Ed)

The key issue was the ability, when actually talking to patients (on the telephone or in person), to 'divorce yourself from what's going on'. Not easy when:

'... your partner's gone off sick or perhaps the manager has decided to move.' (Ed)

Some of these GPs seem able to accept that they are unable to solve every problem and that they are going to have bad days like anyone else:

'There are some days when you're better than others – that's human nature.' (Pat)

'It's being able to say to yourself, "Well that didn't go particularly well, but it's not surprising because I had a, b and c problems at home". We say this to our patients but we don't say it to ourselves. But if the patients get a raw deal, they don't want to know that you had a bad day. I don't know how we can solve that one.' (Sam)

It also helps to be able to switch from one consultation to the next, and not to carry feelings, such as grief, from the previous consultation into the current one (this is part of what Neighbour calls housekeeping or taking care of yourself [2]). However, such feelings are an inevitable part of any interpersonal relationship, including (perhaps particularly) the doctor–patient relationship. Awareness of these factors in oneself and acknowledgement of one's own humanity are noted:

> 'We're human beings and we have to take that into the equation. We're supposed to come in here and be a doctor with no other personal pressures. I don't believe that that's right. I think there are some times when you will be particularly good and there are some times when you won't be particularly good. If that's not allowed to come into the equation, then you're not fit to practise. Sometimes you have a good set of consultations and other times you don't. I think it's affected by what's going on in your own head.' (Sam)

Work and self-awareness

When exploring relating to self, the starting point is insight into personal motivation, in particular understanding the need in oneself to be caring, compassionate, wanted and helpful. The 'liking to be liked' and searching for 'the huge sense of reward' have to be equated with ordinary day-to-day general practice, in which objectivity and realism are essential to provide a balanced service to the patient.

Life experience enters this equation. This is spoken of first in terms of talking about death. Those doctors who have not had intimate experience of death in their own personal life worry that this makes them less helpful in advising and supporting their patients. Although possibly frightening, having had personal meetings with death is seen as useful experience:

> 'I've learnt a lot from that, which I carry into the bereavement situation. I think I know what the feeling is, compared to when I was in my twenties when I had never seen anybody, apart from patients in hospital which don't seem to be the same. They're just bodies, they haven't got families and friends. You have a different attitude when you get into practice, you see the whole family and the children. When there is a bereavement, everybody's crying and upset, and you suddenly realise that this is a man or a woman that's done this, brought these children up, built the house. So there's a change that goes on as you go through life, medicine in particular. I think your own experiences help an awful lot.' (Chaz)

Second, the life experience of the GP varies from year to year, changing the doctor and his or her way of practising medicine. These doctors are aware that their ideas have altered over the years – they report becoming more comfortable in the role, less frightened of uncertainty and more aware of limitations, less likely to be wound up and to feel that it is essential to resolve all conflicts and more likely to reflect on what is really thought to be important, less likely to fall into traps and more likely to have learnt from mistakes.

Experiences of having been a patient are very important to those doctors who have had them. Insights such as loneliness, helplessness and vulnerability are noted, whether the experience as a patient is of childbirth or of personal illness, or of taking members of their own family through illness:

> 'Have you ever been on the other side of a doctor–patient relationship? It's amazing how you suddenly turn into ..., not a quivering lump of jelly, but you're not assertive. You take on a diminutive role, whatever your problem is. You're in a very vulnerable position. I went to see the surgeon with a lump and I'd "got cancer". So I was terrified, and it's amazing. You're like a 10-year-old child and you put total trust in that person, total trust. I couldn't believe it. It gives you an insight into the way people, for even the slightest problems, put you in this very heady position of authority. That's what people expect of you, even if you see it as a trivial matter, "Just a sore throat".' (Ed)

Such personal experiences as a patient can also get in the way when being in the role of a doctor again, particularly if the personal experience as a patient is ongoing:

> 'I was having lots of tests and I knew something was wrong. Somebody comes in and they've got symptoms that sound as if they might be malignant or whatever. You know what you should be asking, but you really want to ask or hear them give the symptoms which are the same perhaps as what you're suffering. Trying to listen to other people's problems, which are very similar to your own, was difficult to carry.' (Tim)

Unsurprisingly, having a family oneself changes many things. The responsibilities of being a parent may increase understanding for, and empathy with, patients, but they also impinge on day-to-day general practice work. They may involve stricter timekeeping to allow for collecting children or other practical issues. Children are occasionally taken on visits and left in the car when there are pressures both at home and at the surgery. They may phone with a crisis in the middle of surgery:

> '... and then you've got the rest of the surgery to finish, when you really want to get on the phone and get sorting. So you try and listen attentively and spend time with the patient, but half your mind is somewhere else.' (Tim)

It may be necessary to:

> '... spend your time at home mothering your kids, and then go to the surgery and have to do it there as well. Though ... skills learnt at the practice are very useful at home managing the family.' (Alex)

Having one's own family and emotional life creates vulnerabilities in the GP. 'What if it was me or my family?' is the question that arises frequently, when for example, as described in Chapter 9, someone the same age as the GP gets cancer or dies suddenly or a child the same age as the general practitioner's child develops schizophrenia or meningitis. It is hard to remain detached and to 'block off', aloof to the implications for your own mortality or that of your family:

> 'I felt very sad recently, and it got to me a little bit, when a young mum developed abdominal cancer. She had a family, similar ages to my children. I think it sort of hit home that these things can happen to any of us. I got quite involved with the family and it was difficult when she died. I did feel emotional and it did hit home.' (Lee)

Self-awareness involves knowing one's own limitations. This includes understanding that:

> 'There is a finite end to my skills and abilities' (Will)

> 'We are all equipped to deal with some things and not with others' (Don)

and that not knowing all the answers is normal and acceptable. While it can be difficult to accept not curing everyone, and making mistakes from time to time, self-awareness is admitting that doctors:

> '... can't get it right all of the time' (Ed)

and being able to talk about this without feeling a failure or threatened by it:

> 'Often you don't resolve these things. I allow myself self-absolution, because I aim to be right 80% of the time, so I allow myself a little time to fail.' (Ed)

But self-awareness is also realistically assessing strengths, such as listening skills or specific clinical skills:

> 'Certain things I can do very well, certain things I can't do well, and certain things I hate.' (Sam)

Increasing self-awareness, through personal experience, through relating to self, to family, to colleagues and to patients, is an integral part of the growth of the GP from novice to experienced practitioner, and inevitably affects the ability to undertake listening work. Also integral to this growth is knowledge of self-limitation through developing understanding of both conscious competence and conscious incompetence in general practice work.

In this chapter, I have been describing doctors' perceptions of the boundaries they draw between work and personal life. Their degree of attachment or involvement with their patients is influenced by factors both in their patients and in themselves, including their life experience and their level of self-awareness. Increasing the latter, it has been suggested,[3] can improve doctors' clinical care and increase their satisfaction with work, relationships and themselves. In the final chapter of this section, I further explore aspects of the doctors' self. A degree of overlap between Chapters 10 and 11 is inevitable.

References

1   Mead N, Bower P (2000) Patient-centredness: a conceptual framework and review of the empirical literature. *Fam Pract.* **51**: 1087–110.

2   Neighbour R (2004) *The Inner Consultation* (2e). Radcliffe Publishing, Oxford.

3   Novack D, Suchman A, Clark W *et al.* (1997) Calibrating the physician: personal awareness and effective patient care. *JAMA.* **278**: 502–9.

11

Work and self: adequacy and sincerity

General practice is:

'A lonely thing to do involving very intimate relationships.' (Lee)

It is also:

'So unpredictable. You don't know what is going to come in the door next.' (Phil)

Some doctors have difficulty, or limits, with certain issues – examples given include poorly children, termination of pregnancy, questions about their personal life, patients who are angry and Monday mornings generally. As a result, listening work may be altered and effects created on the doctor's self, such as guilt, feelings of insincerity or fears of inadequacy. Some of these effects are explored in this chapter.

Satisfaction and adequacy

The satisfaction of being a GP centres, for these doctors, on aspects of encounters with patients. This might involve knowing a patient as an 'almost friend', helping someone through a major life event such as obtaining ill health retirement, enabling someone to start to recognise and manage their problems, or 'feeling chuffed' when treatment works. Satisfaction may come from working with individuals or with families:

'Once people want to pour their heart out to you, they are opening up and giving you an awful lot of their own privacy and their personality and their life. It's a great privilege to sit there and listen.' (Adam)

'One of the things I find most interesting and most rewarding about general practice is involvement with individuals as part of a group, particularly the family group. I'm aware of conflicts and other issues that they may not be aware I know directly. I know something about how they tick, why they've got this problem, what's behind it. That all assembles a picture of somebody in society and in life and enables me to be in a very privileged position.' (Lew)

Being thought of as approachable, helpful and part of the family are also seen as important. Words used to describe this satisfaction include *useful, interesting, fascinating, rewarding* and *humbling*; the latter in the context, first, of the perceived responsibility of being important in people's lives as the local doctor and, second, of being given credit, seen as unearned, for things that are 'just part of the job'.

As has been noted, these GPs also speak of enjoying making unusual difficult diagnoses and undertaking the more practical, hands-on, parts of the job, whilst noting that these aspects do not form a major part of the workload (*see* Chapter 5). Several doctors commented on the need to have areas of interest within general practice in order to avoid stagnation. Examples given were occupational health, hospital attachments, research, teaching and training, management and medical politics. Others noted that different things have provided satisfaction at different stages in their careers, particularly learning how to enjoy family life and using skills from work in the family context (such as listening skills in managing teenagers).

Some aspects of job satisfaction create dilemmas, such as treating someone who is dying or making a clever diagnosis of cancer:

'Just as she was going, she said, "My tummy's been bloated recently". I almost let her get out of the door and in the end I said, "Let's have a little feel of that". She had a cancer, absolutely huge. I got so excited about that, even though I like her a lot and I was sad that she has it because she has a lot on her plate. Even so, this excitement of having a medical condition to sort out got the better of me and I enjoyed it a lot. To enjoy someone's real physical problem is an odd thing. I really felt for her. But I enjoy cancer care, although it is sad at the end. I enjoy going through the stages with a patient, more on a clinical basis, although I do get involved with them.' (Lee)

Within the context of a job seen as generally worthwhile and satisfying, there are inevitably times and situations which appear less worthwhile and satisfying. A long on-call day may be tedious, with little recollection of individual patients and no feeling of achievement:

'The job is never boring, it pays well, and the sense of reward is huge a lot of the time. Some of the demands and the pain are also, I suspect, substantially greater than in other jobs.' (Tom)

Feeling satisfied or dissatisfied as a GP seems to be closely linked to feeling adequate or inadequate in the role. The recurrent fear is of not coping:

'It's usually a feeling of inadequacy. I feel, "Oh gosh I'm not equipped for this, I can't cope". But one does. Although I've been doing it for 15 years now, you always think the next patient who rings up will be the one you're not going to cope with. So it's more of a fear, not so much that they put you in a situation, but that you're not equipped to deal with it. But usually you do manage to find the answer. More and more, I know my limitations.' (Tim)

Feelings of inadequacy or failure are frequently induced in these doctors by their patients, who may have unrealistic expectations or be excessively demanding. Examples include patients who cannot be cured or who do not respond to treatment:

'Whatever I do, I just can't get anywhere. She's quite frustrating. I end up just feeling quite useless really.' (Pete)

'I'm struggling. You come up with suggestions and, "Oh no, we've done that, it didn't work". She's a very, very difficult patient. I quite often feel completely at a loss.' (Paul)

'I feel a failure if I can't answer his questions. Perhaps he doesn't expect me to be in a position to answer them anyway.' (Adam)

'No matter what I do, I can't make them any better and I feel a bit of a failure.' (Chaz)

'I feel a complete failure but I have to be realistic. She's not going to stop drinking.' (Phil)

Similarly, patients may know more than their doctor, a situation thought to be increasingly common in this age of information. They may ask to be referred to another health professional for a condition which the GP feels competent to treat, or they may insist on being managed by the GP, who may feel that care could be better provided by someone else. They may choose the GP as the person to give them sympathy and support:

'You're the only person I can talk to.' (Will)

Either way, doctors can be left feeling inadequate, uncomfortable or hopeless.
Self-imposed personal expectations, which are perhaps sometimes unrealistic, also occur:

> 'Everybody wants to maintain a high level of quality and if you are not able
> to maintain that quality, you get upset about it and feel bad about it.' (Ed)

These doctors have bad days, get tired, operate below par some of the time
and then feel guilty. Feelings of not coping, of limitations, of not knowing
enough, of being unable to cure or solve some problems are all part of being
an experienced GP, as is learning to live with mistakes and failure. The three
most common areas are, first, understanding that some patients will choose to
change to a different doctor within a partnership (or occasionally at another
surgery). This is a normal part of general practice and is thought generally,
over time, to be a two-way process. Unfortunately, it may leave the GP from
whom the patient has switched feeling guilty, not knowing why this switch
has occurred and thinking, 'Where have I gone wrong?' and, 'How could I
have handled it differently?'. The second area is that of not giving patients
enough time or cutting them off, of not listening or not listening hard
enough, or of spotting a lead and choosing to ignore it for whatever reason
(as discussed in Chapters 2 and 3). Third, there is living with, and learning
from, the major mistake which may occur during a career:

> 'There are times when things go badly wrong and you think, '"Oh my
> God". You seriously question your clinical skills. "Am I doing the right
> job?" All this sort of business. Having experienced two or three of those in
> the not too distant past, I think that overall I do feel my skills are adequate,
> but it's fairly fragile, it's fairly fragile. You really feel very fragile, very
> vulnerable, very threatened, very self-questioning and all the rest of it.
> Most of the time you probably don't know whether you are doing the best
> you possibly could or whether you've met the patient's needs and
> objectives. You just assume that you have.' (Will)

The ability of each GP to cope and to handle these inevitable feelings of
inadequacy varies from doctor to doctor, and from week to week, and
changes throughout the working lifetime. Almost all these doctors have given
this some thought:

> 'I'm a bit of a perfectionist and that's a problem because there's no way you
> can keep 100% up to date with all the skills that you learnt. Frequently I

question my ability, "Have I done this right, am I confident that this is what I should be doing in this situation now?". Some weeks it's worse than others and I think, "I should pack this up, its not right for me to be treating these people". Then I say to myself, "Don't be ridiculous, you haven't killed anybody". (Vic)

'When I'm in a situation where I feel I've been inadequate, I look at what I've done or not done and say, "What can I learn from this, could I have done it any differently?". If you know that really you've still done your best, then you don't feel so bad. At the end of the day, you live with it, because you know that you can't be all things to all people. When I was a young doctor, if somebody came to me with a problem, I automatically presumed that it was up to me to solve that problem. I think I'm better at understanding my own limitations and knowing and accessing people with other skills.' (Rick)

Being aware of having particular skills with certain conditions or types of people, such as neurological illnesses or diabetes, and having areas of less confidence, such as depression or dealing with drug addicts, is seen as part of this coping, using colleagues' expertise as necessary. Similarly, being an effective practitioner involves knowing personal strengths (conscious competence) and weaknesses (conscious incompetence).

Sincerity (or feeling false)

All these doctors have been in their jobs for at least five years (some for more than 25 years). Despite this, there is reflection, discussed above, on the theme of adequacy and coping with the day-to-day business of being a GP. This reflection comes as much from doctors who have been in post more than 25 years as from those in post nearer to five years. Similarly, feeling false or insincere with patients seems to be a consideration for these doctors at all stages in their career. Having said that, it is important to note that any insincerity or falseness reported here is apparent more as a feeling and a worry than an attempt to be deceitful or anything other than helpful to patients.

The reflections of these doctors on sincerity fall into five areas. The first and simplest is the acknowledgement that it is a great relief to go on holiday, maternity leave or study leave, allowing someone else to pick up the pieces and take on the pressures of patient care. Similarly, however dedicated the GP, being on-call or duty doctor is a burden.

The second area is described in the following quotation:

'You do need to have a sort of repertoire of situations you can deal with when people come to see you. You almost feel a bit like a tape recorder really, when you speak to somebody and very often you are saying very similar things. It does tend to get a bit like that I think.' (Ben)

This might involve having an 'anxiety' speech, a 'starting the pill' speech or a 'sore throat but no tonsillitis' speech, for example. These speeches contain broadly similar content but are varied for each patient's individual situation. The words *tape recorder* and *autopilot* were mentioned a few times, but generally in the same breath as integrity and:

'... always doing your best to deal with that problem for that patient at that time.' (Huw)

The third area is concerned with 'putting on a sincere face'. This does not, as was emphasised several times, involve falsehood or lying to patients, but it may involve the doctor feeling false or not quite sincere:

'I feel I'm very false sometimes with patients. I would like them to feel comfortable and guided and supported, but sometimes I know that I'm holding their hand because they'll get something out of it but there is a bit of insincerity from me. Several times, patients have said, "Thank you, we know you have done all you could and you did a fantastic job" but I didn't really feel that I did. I could have done more or handled it in a better way. Sometimes I feel guilty that perhaps inside I don't feel what my outside is telling the patient.' (Adam)

This feeling false, which was shared by several doctors, is not seen as insincerity but more as:

'Just trying to move people along a bit.' (Ed)

One GP, describing the need to occasionally pretend to be very religious in order to help, was quite clear that occasionally he is acting or performing, though only in the patient's best interests:

'I'm an actor. It's a con as far as I'm concerned but it's so beneficial to the patient. When I go out of the room, I think, "What a con". I say that to myself, as I'm going to the car, because I'm sure that actors feel that as well when they get off the stage and they've reverted back to being themselves.

It's a play, it's an act. You're doing something that you know is going to be helpful but you're not so sure whether you believe it.' (Chaz)

Fourth, there is the problem of coping with patients the GP does not like:

'It's always difficult if you don't like the person, and of course you can't like everybody. That's when it becomes a challenge. There are several patients that really I can't stand the sight of, literally. How do I handle that? I suppose you 'look at the ceiling and think of England' is a somewhat glib answer, but it's along those lines. You certainly listen, you try and be pleasant with them. You sit and listen to them often ranting and raving at you about things. It comes to an end and they go, and you just hope it's not going to be soon before they come back and visit you. You're obviously not being sincere, but trying to portray sincerity when it really isn't there. Oddly enough, they don't pick that up.' (Steve)

Lastly, there is the issue of maintaining sincerity when the GP is under pressure for external reasons, and when his or her mind is 'there but not there'. Examples given include going on holiday tomorrow, a meeting to rush off to or a telephone call to be made:

'That's usually when I'm stressed, not through work but through home. I've got a busy week, I'm rushing here, there and everywhere with the children, maybe my (spouse) is working away. I'm under pressure. Then I'm thinking, "I can't be bothered with this, let's just do the minimum that's satisfactory". If I'm not happy with what I've done, I tell them to come back. I do try and sit back and say, "Look, somebody's come to consult you, you've got to give them the business". ... You're maybe not quite being sincere.' (Vic)

In concluding, it is important to state again that although these doctors have clearly reflected at times on their feelings of sincerity, insincerity and feeling false (one even describing himself as 'a bluffer'), this is invariably described within the overall context of a professional, concerned and caring GP–patient relationship.

In this section, I have explored perceptions of boundaries and the doctor's self in primary care. Judging boundaries or interpersonal limits is influenced by structure (the situation) and agency (the individuals involved – both patients and doctors). I have summarised these factors in Box 11.1. They both influence and are influenced by the doctor's self, vary in their importance between doctors and over time, and can influence outcome. For example, liking in the doctor–patient encounter influences patient satisfaction.[1] Similarly, the doctor's personal experience of illness (the 'wounded healer') affects encounters with patients.[2,3] In the concluding chapters of this book, I will consider these issues further by discussing some of the themes arising from each section.

Box 11.1   Factors in the doctor's self influencing judgements of interpersonal distance in doctor–patient encounters

- Ability to prioritise patient's problems
- Guilt, for example booking a double appointment and so seeing fewer patients
- Irritation with aspects of the job
- Tension at having to create limits and so not meeting perceived needs
- Ability to separate professional and personal self
- Fear of not coping and feeling inadequate
- Self-imposed unrealistic expectations
- Current mood
- Need to be liked
- Personal life experience, for example bereavement, being a patient or a parent
- Feelings towards individual patients, for example of attachment or dislike
- Fear of inappropriate emotional attachment from patient to doctor
- Pre-existing relationship, for example knowing patient socially or through school
- Identifying with patients, for example same age and sex

References

1   Hall J, Horgan T, Stein T *et al.* (2002) Liking in the physician–patient relationship. *Patient Educ Couns.* **48**:69–77.

2   Rippere V, Williams R (eds) (1985) *Wounded Healers*. Wiley, Chichester.

3   Jackson S (2001) The wounded healer. *Bull History Med.* **75**:1–36.

12

Listening as work in primary care

The three sections of this book have provided a detailed insight into the day-to-day world of doctors in primary care working in a semi-rural area in the north of England at the start of the twenty-first century. In this chapter, I review themes from the three sections and discuss some of the questions raised. The book concludes with a postscript.

Stories and journeys in listening work

In Chapter 1, I suggested that stories, such as the narrative accounts of 'doing' listening work in everyday general practice on which this book is based, are important in understanding in medicine. I also noted Neighbour's helpful description of the consultation as a journey.[1] This metaphor can usefully be extended to include the ongoing doctor–patient relationship in primary care.

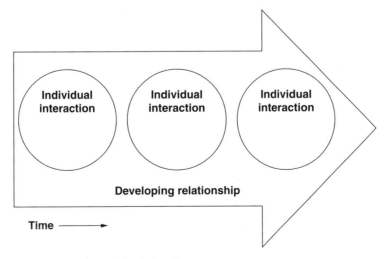

Figure 12.1   General model of the GP–patient encounter.

This relationship is built on cumulative listening work and in primary care this takes place in everyday interactions, mostly face-to-face consultations, between doctors and their patients. This is represented in Figure 12.1. Recurrent or cumulative interactions both build the relationship and in themselves form a journey. This journey, the developing and ongoing doctor–patient relationship, has been central to family medicine for a long time but is under-represented in the current literature of primary care. This journey also points to doctors' own journeys through life and through their careers. The accounts in Section 3 suggest that doctors in primary care need to understand something of their own self and their personal journey (for example, feelings of inadequacy or guilt) because, without such self-understanding, their listening work with patients may be affected.

Levels of listening work in primary care

In considering listening in the work of these primary care doctors, I have described the 'listening loop', defined as a definite period of listening by the GP within the interaction, generally separate to hearing the patient's initial story. This model of listening provides focus on an important moment of judgement within the GP–patient interaction (whether or not to set off into listening in response to a patient's cue), raising the issue of limits to listening work. Choice involves power, with consequent opportunity for resistance. For example, the doctor's judgement may be to maintain a clinical gaze that is limited to objective and biomedical factors, rather than to engage in listening work, by going down the loop and allowing more subjective issues to emerge.

Work and relationship consequent to listening have been discussed. Pastoral work (being available for reliable supportive care not concerned with clinical medicine) is integral to the practice of these doctors. Holding work built on cumulative listening over time (a trusting, constant, reliable GP–patient relationship that is concerned with support, giving time and keeping people going) has been described.

Lastly, the pragmatic negotiation of boundaries and limits to listening and relating perceived by these doctors in their everyday work, both with their patients and in themselves, has been outlined. These factors framing listening work include structure (such as organisation of time in an individual surgery or within a practice) and agency (such as limits to encounters set by doctors, ways in which limits are challenged and varied, and the effect of this work on the doctor's self). These ideas are presented in Figure 12.2, which develops Figure 12.1 – although the diagram shows a listening loop in every interaction, I think this is unlikely to be the case in everyday practice!

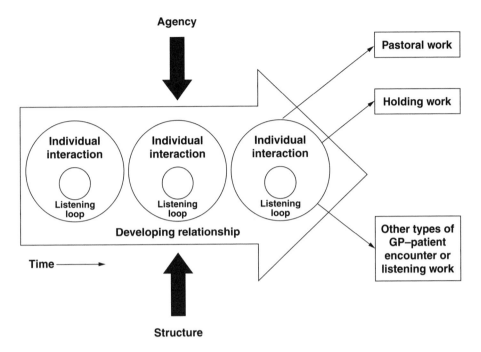

Figure 12.2   Overview: listening as work in the GP–patient encounter.

As we have seen, listening by doctors in primary care can be seen at several different levels, both with patients and in other contexts – I have summarised this listening work in Box 12.1. Some of this communication can be learnt, some is more attitudinal (for example, valuing listening work) and hence harder to teach. Some perhaps cannot be fully understood outside an ongoing relationship between a patient and an experienced GP. Some involves support for doctors as they undertake listening work, an area which is essential but which I have not explored.

Box 12.1   Levels of listening work in primary care

Listening with patients:
- As a set of communication skills at the start of the interaction, to hear the initial story
- As a conscious awareness of, and alertness for, cues being presented by the patient, both at the start of and during the interaction
- As a set of communication skills during the interaction, to allow a 'loop' of listening to occur, either as part of an ongoing narrative or as a simple therapeutic act in itself

- As a set of communication skills to complete an individual interaction and, if necessary, to plan for further listening in future interactions
- As a cumulative act that establishes and builds relationship, both within an individual interaction and as part of an ongoing encounter
- As part of an attitude that values time spent listening
- As part of conversations with significant others which act to witness, validate or legitimate reality for individuals and help order their place within the world

Listening in other contexts:
- As part of interacting with colleagues, family and others
- As part of self-awareness, and relating to oneself
- As part of recognition of various pressures that elicit judgements and choices from doctors with consequent setting of limits on listening in the reality of everyday work
- As part of support for doctors from colleagues, family and others

The typology of holding work in primary care described in Chapter 6 forms a continuum, from long-term continuous holding, via long-term episodic holding, to interim holding. Similarly, a continuum of clinical encounters (Box 12.2) can be used to link this typology into everyday general practice.

Box 12.2   A continuum of clinical encounters

- Routine single interactions
- Brief series of interactions around one or more particular problems
- Interim holding – seeing someone regularly for up to one year for support, reassurance or working through a life event
- Co-ordinating and managing severe physical illness, such as cancer or multiple sclerosis
- Long-term monitoring of chronic physical illness, such as hypertension, diabetes
- Long-term holding – continuous or episodic – support with little active treatment or investigation

---

In a study of family physicians' experience of clinical encounters, Miller[2] described four encounter types.

- Routine encounters: for minor infections, trauma, reassurance or examination.

- Dramas: complications, difficulties or troubles associated with crises, bad news, family discord or insoluble diagnoses.
- Transition ceremonies: 'schedule busters' filled with surprise challenges such as presenting a new diagnosis of chronic disease.
- Maintenance ceremonies: such as well-child or pre-natal care visits or visits containing management of chronic care needs.

Holding appears to be a maintenance ceremony in this typology because patients described as needing a long-term holding relationship clearly have chronic care needs. Miller[2] suggests that if a doctor engaged in a clinical interaction can identify where this interaction lies in a framework, typology or continuum (such as those discussed above), it may promote efficiency, satisfaction and understanding of decision making concerning clinical encounters. This suggestion implies conscious competence in interaction identification during an interaction, and fits well with the conscious competence required for judgements about listening work noted earlier (for example, spotting cues, choosing to listen or not to listen within an interaction, or choosing to use holding as a management strategy).

Continuity of care and listening work

The 'knowledge and trust engendered by repeated contacts' between patients and doctors[3] are apparent in the accounts of holding in Section 2 and also in the literature of general practice. Fugelli[4] described six 'basic instincts of general practice', the first two of which are personal doctoring and continuity of care. Continuity of care has been called 'the most important prerequisite' for personal care[5] and is regarded as important by both patients and doctors.[6,7] If a patient looks to a particular practitioner as their most valued source of care, the nature and quality of the contacts are more important than their frequency,[8,9] and the patient will be willing to wait to see a particular doctor or to travel a greater distance.[10] Continuity of care leads to increased trust and patient satisfaction[11] and to greater accumulated knowledge by GPs of their patients[12] which saves time.[13] However, work is being redistributed within primary healthcare teams[14] and there are fears that both continuity of care and personal care are currently being eroded.[15]

Continuity of care for a period of time is a prerequisite for a holding relationship and is implicit in the descriptions of pastoral work given by these doctors, all of whom have been in practice for more than five years. Despite these factors, no firm conclusions can be drawn from this book concerning the place of continuity or personal doctoring in listening work. It may be that being in the position of a GP is enough to be trusted and asked for 'reliable supportive care' without the necessity for the cumulative listening that builds relationship.

Legitimate listening work in primary care

> At the present day, the doctor has largely taken the place of the confessor. (Anonymous 1899)[16]

For some years, GPs have been described as 'medicine's parish priests'[17] or 'the new clergy'.[18] The Archbishop of Canterbury noted in 1996 that:

> ... many general practitioners are bombarded with demands upon their time and the desire for pills for every ill. Once people who felt fed up or mildly depressed talked to their neighbours, to their older relatives or even to their parish priest. Today they are much more likely to go to their GP instead. In many cities neighbours no longer talk to each other, families are dispersed and increasingly fragmented, and parish priests are fewer in number. In this post-modern environment of social fragmentation, the GP seems to be the only one left to listen to people's troubles and even to hear their 'confessions'. Yet a busy surgery was never intended to carry such a burden.[19]

Jung[20] observed that 'patients force the psychotherapist into the role of the priest and expect and demand that he shall free them from distress'. The same sentence could as easily apply to family doctors as to psychotherapists. The first-generation psychotherapists were aware of the continuity of their procedures with the religious soul-care of priests or spiritual directors.[21] Freud[22] described psychoanalysis as 'pastoral work in the best sense of the words'. Snow (1967) argued that:

> Modern life is becoming entirely deprived of any sense of community. There is no wise man, the religion which was preached is no longer listened to. We have to find people who are respected, who are on the spot, who are sensible and who can perform some kind of function of religion. I believe that general practitioners have always understood this. ... How are we going to continue and possibly develop this particular spiritual and social function of general practitioners?[23]

From the narratives in this book, it would appear that the suggested social function of the GP is being undertaken, at least at some level, by these doctors.

They make no claims to be wise men or women and quite emphatically do not identify the religious or spiritual in what they do (in this book, I have not presented the evidence which was gathered supporting this latter assertion). However, they are 'on the spot', balancing the claims of scientific medicine and offering both a skilled technical service and a relational, pastoral role.

The dilemma of balancing is not new for family doctors. The following comes from a RCGP symposium on 'Society and its General Practitioners' in 1967:

> The doctor is compelled to adopt a dual role. He both prescribes physical remedies and acts as a counsellor on personal and social problems; and in the latter capacity he can hardly avoid passing judgement on issues that are moral rather than medical, and on which, as he would be the first to agree, he can claim no special competence.[24]

These doctors identify pastoral listening work as part of their normal role. They may not immediately name it as 'pastoral', but they can define it in general terms, understand their patient's expectations and needs for an 'experienced friend', regard it as appropriate, note that it occurs frequently in their work and identify the difficulties that it may produce (such as worrying about not getting it right, having no training or being overwhelmed).

Box 12.3   Pastoral and holding work: definitions and issues presented

Pastoral work	Holding work
Definition	
Being available for reliable supportive care not concerned with clinical medicine	Establishing and maintaining a trusting, constant, reliable GP–patient relationship that is concerned not with cure but with support, giving time and keeping people going
Issues presented	
• Family and relationship issues	• Mental health problems (non-acute, non-psychotic)
• Loss and bereavement	
• Lifestyle and social issues	• Loss and bereavement
• Other life events	• Relationship difficulties

I have summarised the definitions of pastoral and holding work described in earlier chapters and the needs that patients are thought to present in Box 12.3. It is apparent that pastoral issues are to do mostly with life events, relationship issues and general unhappiness. Holding overlaps with these but includes non-acute mental illness. Both pastoral and holding work, for these doctors, span the boundary between non-acute, non-psychotic mental illness, which may be seen as biomedical in nature, and general well-being and quality of life issues, seen as psychosocial. The question arises as to what extent undertaking pastoral listening work and attending to these psychosocial issues and subjective pathologies is legitimate work for the GP.

Professional role definitions clearly imply that pastoral work is part of the doctor's role in primary care. For example, in the *European Definition of General Practice/Family Medicine* noted in Chapter 1,[3] general practice 'has a unique consultation process, which establishes a relationship over time, through effective communication between doctor and patient,' and 'deals with health problems in their physical, psychological, social, cultural and existential dimensions', utilising 'the knowledge and trust engendered by repeated contacts'. Applying medical science to a disease process is only one part of patient care, which should also address the illness (the social model) and the hopes, fears, feelings and expectations of the patient.[25] All aspects of human existence are the legitimate concerns of the GP provided that they are presented as a problem by the patient.[26] John Fry, writing in the late 1970s,[27] suggests that the GP will have 'special responsibilities as a personal and family friend, philosopher, and confidant as well as medical advisor'. Similarly, general practice has been described as the 'only medical speciality that is interested in people first and disease second. GPs are interested in personality, family patterns, and the effect of these on the presentation of symptoms as much as in the diseases themselves'.[28]

The definition of pastoral work in primary care given earlier is 'being available for reliable supportive care not concerned with clinical medicine'. That such work takes place in everyday practice is clear from both the present accounts and the literature;[29–34] one study found the doctor's main task was counselling and emotional support in 12.9% of consultations.[33] It has even been argued, on the basis that an interaction with a GP does not happen in isolation and involves a complex interplay between different aspects of a person's life, that all consultations have a psychosocial component.[34] Although this pastoral work is an implicit part of the role definitions discussed above, it is not generally explicitly named. A clearer focus in the literature of primary care would help understanding of this part of the GP's work (for example, the WONCA definition[3] above does not discuss or make clear the meaning and implications of the word *existential*).

That some of these doctors did not immediately identify being pastoral, even though they report undertaking such listening work, is in line with the focus of their training in the identification and management of clinical pathology.[35,36] Additionally, a minority of these doctors felt pastoral work was not a good or appropriate use of their time. Their views echo those of an urban questionnaire study in which GP respondents saw themselves as having a bio(psycho) focus, allotting low priority to the 'social' aspect of their work.[37] Similarly, in *Choosing Talking Therapies?*,[38] a publication aimed at 'anyone who is depressed or unhappy, or who has emotional problems they cannot sort out on their own', the UK Department of Health uses an evidence-based guideline[38] to give the following explanation:

> Talking therapies involve talking and listening. Most of us want somebody to talk to, who listens and accepts us, especially when we are going through a bad time. Sometimes it is easier to talk to a stranger than to relatives or friends. Some therapists will aim to find the root cause of your problem, some will help you to change your behaviour or negative thoughts, while others aim simply to support you. Therapists are trained to listen attentively. . . . (they) can help you through a crisis or difficult patch in your life.[38]

The talking therapies suggested are counselling, cognitive behaviour therapy and psychoanalytical and psychodynamic therapies. 'The people you are likely to see on the NHS who may offer talking therapies'[38,39] are listed as community psychiatric nurses, counsellors, psychiatrists, psychologists, psychotherapists and 'others', such as social workers and occupational therapists. There is no mention of, or value attached to, the listening work of GPs, whose role is described solely as referral to these other agencies. This is despite the overlap between these doctors' perceptions of their everyday listening work and the work of the talking therapists outlined above. For example, the latter have as an area of work 'adjustment to life events',[39] which is an integral part of the GP's role (*see* Box 12.3 above). This omission may be because the role of the GP as talking therapist is little defined with a poor evidence base compared with specialist psychological treatments, where there have been significant, well-researched therapeutic developments.[40,41] Although these GPs do not see themselves as 'amateur counsellors', they are clear that their listening work complements that of the talking therapists listed above – liaising with and referring to such therapists is part of their role, but undertaking listening work (or talking therapy) themselves is an equally important and potentially therapeutic part of their work.

So what is legitimate listening work for doctors in primary care? I have noted the social role suggested for family doctors in a fragmenting society in which they are on the spot, respected and sensible,[23] perhaps functioning as experienced friends capable of attending to all aspects of human existence.[26] I have outlined the long-standing dilemma, or dual role, this creates for GPs, evident in this book, in the literature and in professional role definitions, of balancing 'prescribing physical remedies'[24] with pastoral work, for which they can claim 'no special competence'.[24] Listening as work in everyday primary care may be seen as a process which has the aim of revealing and managing problems, be they biomedical and objective or less clinical and more subjective. These doctors generally see attending to subjective pathology (such as pastoral and holding work) as a core and legitimate part of their role. However, this listening role may not be explicitly named by them, is not fully defined in the profession's view of its role, and is not generally recognised within the wider NHS, in part because of a poor evidence base.

Listening and the importance of conversations

Listening work in medicine is driven by the need to undertake clinical encounters and build professional relationships. Although these relationships vary from patient to patient and from situation to situation, cumulative listening builds relationship and listening work in each doctor–patient interaction builds the doctor–patient relationship. But the significance of listening is wider than this. In discussing the sociology of marriage, Berger and Kellner argued that:

> ... one converses one's way through life. ... The reality of the world is sustained through conversations with significant others.[42]

The doctor–patient relationship may be one of the significant relationships in the wider community, outside marriage, which is socially legitimated and meaningful for members of society in the UK. The GP will qualify as a 'significant other' for many patients, though clearly the doctor–patient relationship cannot be equated to marriage in terms of significance. Conversations with significant others may act to validate the world of the individual and his or her place within that world:

> Every individual requires the ongoing validation of his world, including crucially the validation of his identity and place in this world, by those few who are truly his significant others. ... In everyday life, the principal method employed is speech. In this sense it is proper to view the individual's relationship with his significant others as an ongoing conversation.[42]

Listening in conversation with significant others can both establish relationships and become part of the ordering of reality for individuals. Talking
through experiences, witnessed by a significant other, may make them real.
This book provides numerous examples of experiences being talked through,
including bereavement, illness and difficulties with relationships. It can be
argued that humanity, and each community, needs such witnesses. The
psychotherapist Paul Fleischman has described 'witnessed significance':

> Patients will talk about the need to be seen, known, responded to,
> confirmed, appreciated, cared for, mirrored, recognised, identified. This
> need is prototypically fulfilled by parents, and by the nurturing strata of
> society – grandparents, teachers, doctors, priests. It corresponds to the
> needs written about as 'early infantile narcissism' in psychoanalytical
> writing. The need is universal. Depending on the vicissitudes in any one
> individual's life, fulfilment may be sought in aching and raging despera-
> tion, or in calm and confident relatedness, but the need is more than a
> childhood deficiency helped by soothing or holding. I call this need:
> witnessed significance.[43]

The GP who works to listen over time, and hence build a relationship, can be
seen as offering 'witnessed significance' to those patients who search for such
human 'honest communication and trusting confidence':[43]

> The key roles of the general practitioner are firstly to serve as interpreter
> and guardian at the interface between illness and disease; and secondly to
> serve as a witness to the patient's experience of illness and disease.[26]

In the context of medical communication, this has in part been described as
legitimation ('specifically communicating acceptance and validation of the
patient's emotional experience'[44]). Although none of the doctors interviewed
have made such claims for themselves, they clearly identify listening as part
of their work and the necessity to take into account far more than just
physical illness. They also acknowledge that, for their patients, they represent a familiar face in the community, often the only person easily available
and accessible, whether the problem is physical or otherwise. At one level,
GPs who undertake this listening work over a period of time build up the
doctor–patient relationship by establishing trust and sharing. At another
level, they may act as an 'empathic witness'[45] or significant other 'walking
with' patients,[46] witnessing the construction and sustaining of reality or of an
illness narrative. Such witnessing may be significant at a particular time or
over a period of time. In *A Fortunate Man*, the Forest of Dean GP, John
Sassall, is described as:

... the objective witness of [his patients'] lives ... the clerk of their records ... He is their own representative. ... He keeps the records so that, from time to time, they can consult them themselves.[47]

The GP may be a 'significant other' in an ongoing relationship, a legitimating person to whom the individual can return. Considering listening through this 'micro-social' focus permits an awareness of the varying nature and significance of the doctor–patient relationship.

Power and legitimate listening work

The judgements these doctors report in their interactions with their patients, particularly concerning legitimate listening work, the patient's subjective issues or pathology and factors influencing these judgements, reflect the inherent power differential in the GP–patient interaction. In the next two sections, I consider these further.

It may be that an individual in need of pastoral listening work ('trustworthy supportive care not concerned with clinical medicine') may both fully understand that this is not a biomedical problem and also feel he has nowhere else to turn for such care that is reliable, free and easily accessible in the community. This need, which the patient perceives as legitimate work for the doctor irrespective of the doctor's definition of work, may be hidden behind a biomedical story. For patients who have non-biomedical or subjective life issues and who 'really have nobody else at all to talk to' (Chris), these doctors see themselves as acting as 'a sort of elder' or 'another family'. Dowrick has described the doctor as a suitable trusted significant person, who may act 'as a third grandmother'.[48] If this is the case, the physical space of the surgery and the social space of the doctor–patient interaction may simply be chosen by the patient as safe, reliable and trustworthy, not specifically as representative of the healthcare system or even requiring the adoption of a sick role to permit entry.

These doctors report that their main tools for this pastoral role are experience and common sense, and that they have had no formal training for it. As a result, the 'competence gap', which some social scientists argue is maintained by the profession's monopoly on medical knowledge,[49,50] is narrowed and the power balance in the relationship altered. This is in contrast to arguments that extending the medical gaze to patients' social and psychological worlds increases medical power and risks medicalising society.[51,52] When faced with problems 'rooted in the realm of the social', GPs report an uncomfortable sense of power being with the patient.[53] Additionally, the power of the patient in primary care is, first, in attending with any pathology, objective or subjective, to which the GP must respond and, second, in the ability to attend the surgery at will and without regard to cost (subject to structural factors like appointment availability). The practitioner's contractual obligation to be there when the patient presents with anything and attends any time forms the context within which the doctor makes judgements and creates boundaries concerning listening work. These are key differences separating the listening work of the GP from that of, for example, nurses or counsellors.

The (macro) level of professional rhetoric and role definition noted earlier[3] implies that listening work is always legitimate. At the everyday (micro) level of the individual interaction, these doctors report responding to their patients' power by making judgements about limiting listening in order to work pragmatically in the constrained time and space of daily practice. Hence the power of the patient to attend in a primary healthcare setting and present a subjective pathology (whether or not sought by the doctor) is met by the power of the doctor to make a judgement (whether or not to listen), rendering the pathology visible or invisible in the encounter and so legitimate or non-legitimate. The GP can choose either to engage in listening work or to resist the patient's presentation of subjective pathology. Evident in these accounts is resistance to the medical gaze not in the surveyed patient but in the surveying doctor, when asked to gaze at subjective pathology by the patient.

Power, boundaries and listening work

Some psychotherapists and counsellors are very firm in maintaining therapist or patient boundaries that are well defined and thought to be therapeutically important.[54,55] The situation is not comparable for these doctors, who generally live in the same community as their patients and may be well-recognised and active members of that community. The blurring of boundaries noted earlier (the consultation over the garden wall, in the supermarket, at the golf club, in the playground or at a child's activity) is part of their everyday general practice. The effect on doctors of this blurring depends on their judgement as to the legitimacy of the interaction – the legitimate interaction is reported to be acceptable and rewarding, the non-legitimate can be embarrassing, awkward and unacceptable, and lead to worries about confidentiality and competence.

Symbolic of this judgement is the doctor's decision on where to live, whether or not to have a physical distance between self (home) and patient (the community served by the practice). A contrast has been described between those doctors who live locally to the practice and judge it legitimate to be interrupted while off duty, and those who prefer the physical boundary of living elsewhere.

Boundary pressures also arise when doctors are seen as patients by these GPs, and from doctors' experiences of being patients themselves. The latter can have a profound effect on a doctor's insight,[56,57] the experience of suffering being 'useful preparation for work in the helping professions'.[58] Bennet[59] suggests that such 'wounded healers' are able to be readily empathic, vulnerable, weak and without masks in their GP–patient relationships and notes that the association of healers with personal weakness or wounds dates back to Greek mythology. However, many medical practitioners have the idea that 'illness is inappropriate for doctors'[60] and this may act as a barrier in their management. Doctors tend to treat themselves and to delay seeking medical help,[61] the healthcare of GPs being 'sketchy at best and dangerous at worst'.[62]

McKevitt and Morgan[63] have described three types of medical encounter that may occur for the 'doctor-as-patient'.

- The patient is in control – the treating doctor acquiesces and continues to relate to the doctor-as-patient as a colleague rather than a patient. The doctor-as-patient may dictate investigations, diagnosis and treatment.
- Like any ordinary patient – this requires some negotiation. The treating doctor may explicitly tell the doctor-as-patient, 'I will treat you like an ordinary patient,' which asserts authority and establishes roles.
- Extraordinary patients, extraordinary needs – this sort of relationship, more advocated than achieved, involves the doctor-as-patient seeing only colleagues experienced in treating medically qualified patients.

These authors go on to observe that:

> ... our data suggest that doctor/patients and the doctors they consult do not simply adopt or fail to adopt an appropriate role. The event raises questions about what kind of doctor to be, what kind of patient to be: for the patient, how to accommodate two apparently contradictory statuses; for the doctor, how to relate to an insider as if he or she were an outsider.[63]

There are clear parallels in Chapter 9 concerning establishing boundaries with both friends as patients and doctors as patients. However, with 'friend friends' as patients, it appears generally acceptable to negotiate firm boundaries. With other doctors, both the negotiations and the practicalities of appropriate investigation and treatment are reported as difficult. The boundary that is being negotiated in these situations is about authority and control. The optimum may be an acknowledged negotiation between the doctor-as-patient and the treating doctor, which leads clearly to the doctor-as-patient being treated 'as an ordinary patient', thus establishing a power differential beneficial to both parties.

It is questionable whether the 'doctor as patient' or the 'friend friend as patient' can ever truly be an 'ordinary patient', either to the giver or the recipient of treatment. The literature is incomplete here. The question arises as to what extent a status or role can be switched or varied within a relationship. Consider this (true) example:

> A GP is called after the expected but slow death of a patient he has got to know well over the years. The daughter, also a regular patient well known to the GP, weeps. The GP is overcome by emotion and they both weep for several minutes, during which time the doctor feels unable to function as a GP. After a little while, order and roles are restored and the doctor is able to carry on. Later, the doctor worries about the 'unprofessional' lapse when he was unable to function as a GP.

When both daughter and doctor are weeping, and the doctor feels 'unable to function as a GP', the interaction may be felt to be person-with-person, rather than doctor-with-patient (with we-the-person rather than we-the-professional[64]). Although the GP worried about adequacy afterwards, he was clearly existentially involved or connected,[65] with no performing or insincerity in the emotion of the situation. Even if the GP had been putting on a performance (as noted in Chapter 11 to occur sometimes – a 'sincere face'), it seems unlikely that this would have been any less an adequate GP–patient interaction. Additionally, whether or not the GP feels the interaction is temporarily person-with-person, it remains an encounter between a patient and a doctor. What changes is power. The power differential inherent in a doctor-with-patient encounter is reduced in a person-with-person encounter, narrowing interpersonal distance and revealing the doctor as self. To what extent is the simple existential presence and humanity of the doctor's self adequate or therapeutic in this situation, removed from professional status, knowledge and training? Perhaps the doctor's apparent powerlessness increases the therapeutic potential of the interaction. For Cassell, attachment in doctor–patient relationships is always reciprocal and exposure of the doctor's self, with consequent alteration in interpersonal distance, power and vulnerability, is an inevitable part of the doctor's role:

> Only another person can empathically experience the experience of a person. In medicine the subjects of experience are the patient and the doctor. Only the physician as a person can empathically experience

the experience of a sick person. *It must be finally accepted, therefore, that there can be no substitute for the physician as a person.*[66] (italics in the original)

Given that there is a continuum from doctor-centredness to patient-centredness in the GP–patient relationship,[30] there may also be a continuum in the roles or statuses that these doctors occupy in that relationship. This continuum ranges from self to doctor to performer, all of which have appeared in this book as part of everyday listening work in primary care. The individual may move position on this continuum during or between encounters, altering interpersonal distance and power. If this is the case, then the language of boundaries and limits is inappropriate. At a given point on the continuum, the individual may be both 'doctor' and 'self', or both 'performer' and 'doctor' at the same time. The distinction is between the physician's human self, the self socialised as a medical professional, and the performance (or 'sincere face') that may be offered to others. This fits with other roles or statuses in our lives (in the overall role of parent, one can be both caring mother and strict authoritarian at the same time).

Doctors vary in their degree of attachment in doctor–patient encounters[66] and the self–doctor–performer continuum highlights resistance by doctors in encounters with patients. Some doctors report maintaining distance by staying in doctor or performer role throughout all encounters with patients, for fear of being overwhelmed or paralysed should their self be revealed or perhaps because, as one of May *et al.*'s respondents asserted, they have 'had quite enough of patients' confidences'.[67] Others establish a physical distance to frame their interpersonal encounters by living away from their patients. For these doctors, to reveal their self narrows the professional distance or perhaps reduces intellectual detachment unacceptably. Performing by the GP emerges as both a method of management, to help patients or move them along, and as a method of resistance, to maintain interpersonal distance between doctor and patient and protect the doctor's self. Again, the individual judges the appropriate method and distance, with consequent effects on the self (such as self-awareness, adequacy and sincerity discussed in Chapters 10 and 11).

This self–doctor–performer continuum also allows attention to focus on the doctor's feelings, not just on those of the patient. It can be seen as running parallel, or alongside, the patient-centred–doctor-centred continuum of Byrne and Long.[30] Being doctor centred may be a doctor's personal or natural consulting style, or the GP may 'perform' as doctor centred in an interaction to benefit the patient. Doctors knowing their position on the continuum at any time, and being able to consciously move along it as needed within or between interactions, may reduce the 'relatively static style of consulting' of the majority of GPs noted by Byrne and Long.[30] The ability to successfully adapt or match communication style to the particular needs of a patient during an interaction (for example, powersharing, directiveness, orientation) has been suggested as an integral part of a skilled helping interaction.[68]

The notion of the 'doctor-as-performer' links to developments over the last almost 50 years described in the literature on the doctor–patient relationship in British general practice.[69] These start with the disinterested clinical gaze of the doctor contemplating the patient's depersonalised body, and move on to construct the doctor's individual self, containing the doctor's mind, which examines the patient's mind. The authors conclude that the body of the doctor, as yet little described, provides a location in which 'the conflict between the personal and the professional can be played out'.[69] This book demonstrates boundaries established by doctors in framing work, both with patients and in themselves. Judgements by doctors delineating boundaries in the personal/professional conflict have been described. Something of the body of the doctor emerges in doctors' experiences as patients and in the physical act of weeping with patients. Additionally, the 'doctor-as-performer' has appeared, suggesting a body that can genuinely weep with patients but also can 'perform', putting on a mask or a 'sincere face' when needed. Thus, as the doctor's self or person has begun to be revealed, so also performing and putting on a mask have emerged as methods of resistance to maintain distance between doctor and patient.

Patient-centredness, legitimate work and the doctor's self

In Chapter 1, I described patient-centredness from the frameworks of Stewart et al.[70] and Mead and Bower.[71] I argued that a more complete understanding of the application of patient-centredness in everyday practice is required. I also noted in Chapter 10 that the subjectivity of the doctor (the doctor's self or person) has been little studied.[71] In contributing to a fuller understanding of these issues, I have, first, highlighted being realistic in the doctor–patient encounter (judgements about embarking on listening in the loop, consideration of organisational, interpersonal and intrapersonal limits). Second, it is clear that patients' subjective pathology is accepted as realistic and legitimate listening work in primary care, both pastoral work in the interaction and developing an ongoing holding relationship. I have suggested that the latter is a patient-centred therapeutic alliance. Third, in the context of the effects of listening work on respondents, something of the doctor's self has been revealed. In addition, I have hypothesised a patient-centred listening role for the GP in legitimating and validating the patient.

As we saw in Chapter 1, patient-centred theory aims to understand the whole person,[70] both biopsychosocial and patient-as-person.[71] Such all-encompassing theoretical ideals are also incorporated into professional role definitions.[3] However, inherent in the patient-centred clinical method[70] is the contradiction between an all-encompassing component ('understanding the whole person' – component 2) and a limiting one ('being realistic' – component 6). Similarly, the wide-ranging *European Definition of General Practice/Family Medicine*[3] contrasts with the priority GPs report giving to the biomedical aspects of a patient's pathology, at the expense of social and psychological factors.[37,67] The same conflict between professional aspiration and practical prioritisation is found in nursing.[72,73]

These contrasts, between the theoretical literature of professions and everyday practice, are also evident in this book – listening work is accepted ideally as central ('We are there to listen' (Tim)) but pragmatic judgements are made in order to work realistically ('I consciously block' (Chris)). This tension, between theory and everyday practice, between the collective approach of a profession and the everyday autonomous activity of individual clinicians,[74] also contrasts with the clear expectations of patients that, alongside technical competence, they require humane doctors with time to care.[75–77]

The 'doctor-as-person' or self frames each encounter between a clinician and a patient and affects its content. Hence, each individual practitioner's level of self-knowledge affects everyday work with patients and colleagues. For example, factors identified within the doctor (see Box 11.1) influence and limit judgements concerning interpersonal distance, as do encounters with patients away from the consulting room. Additionally, other factors have been noted (such as adequacy and sincerity) which are implicit in self-knowledge and raise the possibility of insincerity and consciously performing the role of GP, rather than exposing the doctor's self.

Judgements of pragmatic boundaries again raise the question of limits to legitimate work:

> One of the greatest difficulties facing general practitioners is determining the limit to their field of work.[78]

This book provides evidence both of GPs accepting listening work as legitimate and of limits, influenced by a variety of factors, applied by individual doctors to this work. This tension, between perceived legitimate work and practical limits applied in everyday practice, calls into question the realistic application in primary care of the ideals of patient-centred medicine.

References

1   Neighbour R (2004) *The Inner Consultation* (2e). Radcliffe Publishing, Oxford.

2   Miller W (1992) Routine, ceremony, or drama: an exploratory field study of the primary care clinical encounter. *J Fam Pract.* **34**: 289–96.

3   WONCA (2002) *The European Definition of General Practice/Family Medicine.* The European Society of General Practice/Family Medicine, Europe.

4   Fugelli P (1996) The Patient Europe – calling for the general practitioner. *Eur J Gen Pract.* **2**: 26–9.

5   Fox T (1962) Personal medicine. *Bull New York Acad Med.* **38**: 527–34.

6   Roland M, Mayor V, Morris R (1986) Factors associated with achieving continuity of care in general practice. *J Roy Coll Gen Pract.* **36**: 102–4.

7   Bower P, Roland M, Campbell J *et al.* (2003) Setting standards based on patients' views on access and continuity: secondary analysis of data from the general practice assessment survey. *BMJ.* **326**: 258–60.

8   Freeman G, Hjortdahl P (1997) What future for continuity of care in general practice? *BMJ.* **314**: 1870–3.

9   Freeman G, Walker J, Heaney D *et al.* (2002) Personal continuity and the quality of GP consultations. *Eur J Gen Pract.* **8**: 90–4.

10   Humphreys J, Rolley F (1998) A modified framework for rural general practice: the importance of recruitment and retention. *Soc Sci Med.* **46**: 939–45.

11   Baker R, Mainous A, Gray P *et al.* (2003) Exploration of the relationship between continuity, trust in regular doctors and patient satisfaction with consultations with family doctors. *Scand J Prim Health Care.* **21**: 27–32.

12   Hjortdahl P (1992) Continuity of care: general practitioners' knowledge about, and sense of responsibility toward their patients. *Fam Pract.* **9**: 3–8.

13   Hjortdahl P, Borchgrevink C (1991) Continuity of care: influence of general practitioners' knowledge about their patients on use of resources in consultations. *BMJ.* **303**: 1181–4.

14   Charles-Jones H, Latimer J, May C (2003) Transforming general practice: the redistribution of medical work in primary care. *Soc Health Illness.* **25**: 71–92.

15   Hjortdahl P (2001) Continuity of care – going out of style? *Br J Gen Pract.* **51**: 699–700.

16   Anonymous (1899) The doctor in the pulpit. *BMJ.* **i**: 1549.

17   Munro A (1999) Reformation? *Br J Gen Pract.* **49**: 594–5.

18   Heenan C, cited in Hunt J (1969) Religion and the family doctor. *J Roy Coll Gen Pract.* **18**: 199–206.

19   Carey G (1996) *Living with Differences: the Christian church in a post-modern world.* Lecture to the Theology Society by The Archbishop of Canterbury, 7 March 1996. Whitelands College, London.

20   Jung C (1984) *Modern Man in Search of a Soul.* Ark Books, London.

21   Benner D (1988) *Psychotherapy and the Spiritual Quest.* Hodder & Stoughton, London.

22   Freud S (1926) The question of lay analysis. In: Strachey J (ed.) *The Standard Edition of the Complete Psychological Works of Sigmund Freud, Vol 20.* Hogarth Press, London.

23   Snow R (1967) The status of doctors. *Proc Roy Soc Med.* **60**: 153–6.

24   Wootton B (1967) British medical practice as seen through the eyes of a layman. *J Roy Coll Gen Pract.* **79** (supplement 1): 15–24.

25   Royal College of General Practitioners (1996) *The Nature of General Medical Practice. Report from General Practice 27.* Royal College of General Practitioners, London.

26   Heath I (1995) *The Mystery of General Practice.* The Nuffield Provincial Hospitals Trust, London.

27   Fry J, cited in Jones R (1998) Personal medicine and national health. *Fam Pract.* **15**: 189.

28   Davies P (2000) General practitioners' main interest is people. *BMJ.* **321**: 173.

29   Cartwright A (1967) *Patients and Their Doctors.* Routledge & Kegan Paul, London.

30   Byrne P, Long B (1976) *Doctors Talking to Patients.* HMSO, London.

31   Fitton F, Acheson H (1979) *The Doctor–Patient Relationship: a study in general practice.* HMSO, London.

32   Cartwright A, Anderson R (1981) *General Practice Revisited.* Tavistock, London.

33   Winefield H, Murrell T, Clifford J *et al.* (1995) The usefulness of distinguishing different types of general practice consultation, or are needed skills always the same? *Fam Pract.* **12**: 402–7.

34   Hemmings A (1999) *A Systematic Review of Brief Psychological Therapies in Primary Health Care.* Counselling in Primary Care Trust, Staines.

35   Atkinson P (1981) *The Clinical Experience: the construction and reconstruction of medical reality.* Gower, Farnborough.

36   Sinclair S (1997) *Making Doctors: an institutional apprenticeship.* Berg, Oxford.

37   Dowrick C, May C, Richardson M *et al.* (1996) The biopsychosocial model of general practice: rhetoric or reality? *Br J Gen Pract.* **46**: 105–7.

38   Department of Health (2001) *Choosing Talking Therapies?* DoH Publications, London.

39   Department of Health (2001) *Treatment Choice in Psychological Therapies and Counselling. Evidence Based Clinical Practice Guideline.* DoH Publications, London.

40   Cape J, Barker C, Buszewicz M *et al.* (2000) General practitioner psychological management of emotional problems (I): definitions and literature review. *Br J Gen Pract.* **50**: 313–18.

41   Cape J, Barker C, Buszewicz M *et al.* (2000) General practitioner psychological management of emotional problems (II): a research agenda for evidence-based practice. *Br J Gen Pract.* **50**: 396–400.

42   Berger P, Kellner H (1979) Marriage and the construction of reality. In: Berger P (ed.) *Facing Up to Modernity.* Penguin, London.

43   Fleischman P (1990) *The Healing Spirit: case studies in religion and psychotherapy.* SPCK, London.

44   Cohen Cole S, Bird J (1991) Function 2: building rapport and responding to patients' emotions. In: Cohen-Cole S (ed.) *The Medical Interview: the three-function approach.* Mosby, St Louis.

45   Kleinman A (1988) *The Illness Narratives.* Basic Books, New York.

46   McWhinney I (2000) Being a general practitioner: what it means. *Eur J Gen Pract.* **6**: 135–9.

47   Berger J, Mohr J (1967) *A Fortunate Man.* Penguin, London.

48   Dowrick C (1992) Why do the O'Sheas consult so often? An exploration of complex family illness behaviour. *Soc Sci Med.* **34**: 491–7.

49   Friedson E (1970) *Profession of Medicine: a study of the sociology of applied knowledge.* Harper & Row, New York.

50   Waitzkin H (1991) *The Politics of Medical Encounters: how doctors and patients deal with social problems.* Yale University Press, New Haven.

51   Illich I (1976) *Limits to Medicine.* Marion Boyars, London.

52   Chodoff P (2002) The medicalisation of the human condition. *Psychiatric Services.* **53**: 627–8.

53   Wileman L, May C, Chew-Graham C (2002) Medically unexplained symptoms and the problem of power in the primary care consultation: a qualitative study. *Fam Pract.* **19**: 178–82.

54   Hoag L (1992) Psychotherapy in the general practice surgery: considerations of the frame. *Br J Psychotherapy.* **8**: 417–29.

55   Bond T, Alred G, Hughes P (2000) Clinical practice issues. In: Feltham C, Horton I (eds) *Handbook of Counselling and Psychotherapy.* Sage, London.

56   Lupton D (1994) *Medicine as Culture.* Sage, London.

57   Brewer B (1999) Personal view – both sides. *BMJ.* **319**: 1013.

58   Rippere V, Williams R (eds) (1985) *Wounded Healers.* Wiley, Chichester.

59   Bennet G (1979) *Patients and Their Doctors: the journey through medical care.* Baillière Tindall, London.

60   McKevitt C, Morgan M (1997) Illness doesn't belong to us. *J Roy Soc Med.* **90**: 491–5.

61   Allibone A, Oakes D, Shannon HS (1981) The health and healthcare of doctors. *J Roy Coll Gen Pract.* **31**: 728–34.

62   Chambers R (1989) The health of general practitioners: a cause for concern? *J Roy Coll Gen Pract.* **39**: 179–81.

63   McKevitt C, Morgan M (1997) Anomalous patients: the experiences of doctors with an illness. *Soc Health Illness.* **19**: 644–67.

64   Neighbour R (2004) *The Inner Apprentice* (2e). Radcliffe Publishing, Oxford.

65   Suchman A, Matthews D (1988) What makes the patient–doctor relationship therapeutic? Exploring the connexional dimension of medical care. *Ann Intern Med.* **108**: 125–30.

66   Cassell E (1991) *The Nature of Suffering.* Oxford University Press, New York.

67   May C, Dowrick C, Richardson M (1996) The confidential patient: the social construction of therapeutic relationships in general medical practice. *Sociol Rev.* **44**: 187–203.

68   Winefield H, Murrell T, Clifford J *et al.* (1996) The search for reliable and valid measures of patient-centredness. *Psychol Health.* **11**: 811–24.

69   Gothill M, Armstrong D (1999) Dr. No-body: the construction of the doctor as an embodied subject in British general practice 1955–97. *Soc Health Illness.* **21**: 1–12.

70   Stewart M, Brown J, Weston W *et al.* (2003) *Patient-Centred Medicine* (2e). Radcliffe Medical Press, Oxford.

71   Mead N, Bower P (2000) Patient-centredness: a conceptual framework and review of the empirical literature. *Fam Pract.* **51**: 1087–110.

72   Melia K (1987) *Learning and Working: the occupational socialisation of nursing.* Tavistock, London.

73   Davies C (1995) *Gender and the Professional Predicament of Nursing Assessment: an analysis.* Open University Press, Buckingham.

74   Armstrong D (2002) Clinical autonomy, individual and collective: the problem of changing doctors' behaviour. *Soc Sci Med.* **55**: 1771–7.

75   Ware J, Snyder M, Wright R (1984) Defining and measuring patient satisfaction with medical care. *Eval Prog Plan.* **6**: 247–63.

76   Williams S, Calnan M (1991) Key determinants of consumer satisfaction with general practice. *Fam Pract.* **8**: 237–42.

77   Wensing M, Jung H, Mainz J *et al.* (1998) A systematic review of the literature on patient priorities for general practice care. Part 1: description of the research domain. *Soc Sci Med.* **47**: 1573–88.

78   Morrell D (1991) *The Art of General Practice.* Oxford University Press, Oxford.

Postscript: 'I just listened'

In this book, a picture has emerged of a group of doctors going about their everyday practice in the north of England at the start of the twenty-first century. At the end of this journey, the underlying themes threaded throughout are, first, of the value attached to listening work in primary care and, second, of judgements and choices made by doctors in order to manage different levels of listening work.

'I didn't do any medicine, I just listened.'

This comment by a GP registrar, which I overheard in a lunch queue, draws attention to valuing listening work, at a variety of levels, as an integral part of primary care, alongside biomedical and objective pathology. This primary care doctor undertook listening work but did not name, value or recognise it as part of medicine or of a doctor's work. Presumably, listening skills were used in which the doctor is (consciously or unconsciously) either competent or incompetent, and the interaction may or may not have been therapeutic in addressing the patient's psychosocial and subjective issues. In contrast, almost all the accounts which have formed the basis of this book are clear that, alongside attending to organic pathology, 'just listening' is a central part of the work of experienced GPs, irrespective of the content of that listening. Although communication skills are required, 'just listening' is seen not simply as a set of skills but as part of ongoing relationship within and across interactions. It is thought to be a legitimate and potentially therapeutic way to use time in primary care interactions, requiring energy from doctors along with skills, which can be improved by training.

I have described some of the judgements that these experienced doctors make at different levels in their everyday work. Within the interaction, this might involve choosing to use a listening loop or to ignore a cue and risk not addressing important issues for the patient. In the ongoing GP–patient relationship, it might involve choosing to take on holding or pastoral work, or managing relating to 'patients who want to be friends'. In a wider context, it might involve establishing boundaries at different levels (inter- or intrapersonal), influenced by structure (such as appointment times) or agency (such as the need to put on a performance to protect the doctor's self).

These judgements contribute to the management of listening work in primary care, particularly of patients' psychosocial and subjective issues. For example, I have argued that holding work involves person-centred alliances which may be therapeutic. Although largely unnamed, I have identified pastoral work as legitimate listening work taking place regularly in everyday primary care, which balances the skilled technical medical service offered by these doctors. I have discussed literature suggesting that this is a social role, at a societal level, in listening work required of doctors in primary care as 'experienced friends'. Lastly, I have presented evidence that the work of listening in primary care is not well identified or named (and, by inference, is undervalued) by GPs themselves, and by others in the wider NHS.

This last evidence is particularly significant because technological advances, organisational change, resource issues, time pressures, shifting workforce patterns in the NHS and innovations in service provision[1–10] are affecting all work in primary care. These factors frame and put pressure on doctors undertaking and managing listening work in primary care. Parallel questions and choices arise for our society as a whole as to the place of listening work in primary care, social or otherwise,[11] and the value attached to this work. These questions, which go to the heart of the future shape and delivery of primary care, demand attention, not least because our patients' most important requirement of general practice is to have a 'doctor who listens and does not hurry me'.[12]

References

1   Clarkeburn H (1998) Implicit rationing in Britain. *Fam Pract.* **15**: 190–1.

2   O'Connell S (1999) Walk in! Walk out? What *is* it all about? *Br J Gen Pract.* **49**: 765.

3   Florin D, Rosen R (1999) Evaluating NHS Direct. *BMJ.* **319**: 5–6.

4   Akerman F (2000) Is general practice being consigned to history? *BMJ.* **321**: 391.

5   Mechanic D (2001) How should hamsters run? Some observations about sufficient patient time in primary care. *BMJ.* **323**: 266–8.

6   Car J, Sheikh A (2003) Telephone consultations. *BMJ.* **326**: 966–9.

7   Laurant M, Hermens R, Braspenning J *et al.* (2004) Impact of nurse practitioners on workload of general practitioners: randomised controlled trial. *BMJ.* **328**: 927–30.

8   Pickin M, Cathain C, Sampson F *et al.* (2004) Evaluation of advanced access in the primary care collaborative. *Br J Gen Pract.* **54**: 334–40.

9   Chapman J, Zechel A, Carter Y *et al.* (2004) Systematic review of recent innovations in service provision to improve access to primary care. *Br J Gen Pract.* **54**: 374–81.

10   NHS Modernisation Agency (2004) *Physician Practitioners.* NHS Modernisation Agency, London. (www.modern.nhs.uk/cwp/21132/21286/FAQ_physician_ practitioners.pdf) (accessed 10 December 2004).

11   Snow R (1967) The status of doctors. *Proc Roy Soc Med.* **60**: 153–6.

12   Carroll L, Sullivan F, Colledge M (1998) Good health care: patient and professional perspectives. *Br J Gen Pract.* **48**: 1507–8.

Epilogue

Whilst this book was being written, the ways in which British policy makers and general practitioners think about general practices were changing. Ideas about clinical governance and evidence-based practice; changing priorities for healthcare delivery; the increasing concentration of general practice in large group surgeries managed by primary care trusts; and an expanding division of labour in which nurses increasingly took on work formerly done by doctors, all took hold and became important elements of primary care provision, while general practitioners themselves took a step back from out-of-hours care.

So, a number of policy and structural changes occurred that have changed, probably irreversibly, the organisation of doctor–patient relationships in primary care. What has not changed during this period is the central problem that general practitioners face, one that Simon Cocksedge focuses on. This is that many of the problems that are encountered in the everyday consultation are diffuse, with important psychosocial components, and which are the products of the social contexts in which patients are located. All of these figure prominently in this book, as does the ever-growing problem of chronic illness.

The complexity of general practice as a field of medicine means that *listening* to patients and engaging with their affective and social problems remains central to the work of the general practitioner – and also to the primary care and public health nurse, who also encounters these problems in abundance. Ever since Balint[1] general practitioners have regarded these issues as being important. But, increasingly, the means by which the activities of family doctors are assessed focus on quantitative performance indicators and outcome measures. Measuring the performance of general practitioners figures prominently in some of the activities of primary care trusts, but not all that can be counted counts, which is why this book is both interesting and important. It restates the value of *relationship work* in general practice, showing how this work brings with it both responsibilities and problems, but also how it forms part of the solution for many of the real difficulties that people encounter in their everyday lives and bring into the consultation.

Carl May
ESRC Research Fellow and Professor of Medical Sociology
Centre for Health Services Research
University of Newcastle
April 2005

Reference

1 Balint M (1957) *The Doctor, His Patient, and the Illness.* Pitman, London.

Appendices

Appendix I: Methodology

This book is based on a qualitative study in which I interviewed in depth 23 experienced GPs (in practice for at least five years) from one semi-rural area in the north of England. The aim was to expand and further tease out the areas of study in order to identify, describe and understand some of the constituents, and the consequences, of listening work in GP–patient encounters as reported and understood by the doctors interviewed. All the participating doctors had been in practice for at least five years, a cut-off point designed to allow responses firmly rooted in experience of everyday practice. Standard qualitative methods were used for interview analysis,[1–4] the results of which have provided the material for this book. The limitations of this research approach, and hence of conclusions drawn from this work, have been fully explored elsewhere.[3,5] In brief, they cover three areas: the use of qualitative methodology; the restriction of participants to doctors from a relatively small geographical area; and the fact that no patients have been involved. The qualitative approach offers insights which could not be obtained using survey methods. Restricting sampling to a small semi-rural area resulted in an extremely high response rate (23 of 24 eligible GPs being interviewed), but the sample cannot be said to represent British general practice in urban or suburban settings. No conclusions can be drawn about patients' views from the material presented in this book.

References

1   Glaser B, Strauss A (1967) *The Discovery of Grounded Theory: strategies for qualitative research.* Aldine, Chicago.

2   Strauss A, Corbin J (1998) *Basics of Qualitative Research.* Sage, London.

3   Cocksedge S (2003) *Listening as Work – a qualitative investigation into general practitioners' perceptions.* MD thesis. John Rylands University Library, Manchester.

4   Silverman D (ed.) (2004) *Qualitative Research.* Sage, London.

5   Cocksedge S, May C (2005) The listening loop: a model of choice about cues within primary care consultations. *Medical Education.* In press.

Appendix II: Communication skills

In this appendix, I reproduce (with thanks to, and permission from, doctors Silverman, Kurtz and Draper) the basic framework, the expanded framework and the communication process skills of the Calgary–Cambridge Guide. This lists all the communication skills with which we hope to equip our medical students by the time they graduate from the University of Manchester! An outline of this material is at: www.skillscascade.com.

The basic framework of the medical interview

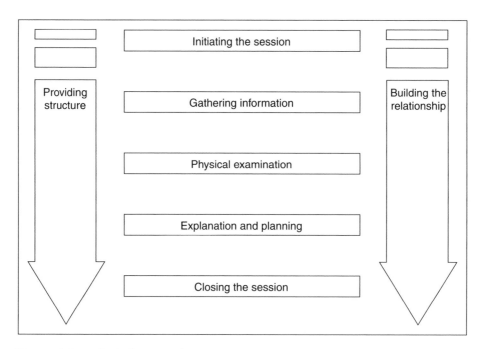

Figure A2.1   Basic framework.

The expanded framework of the medical interview – tasks and objectives

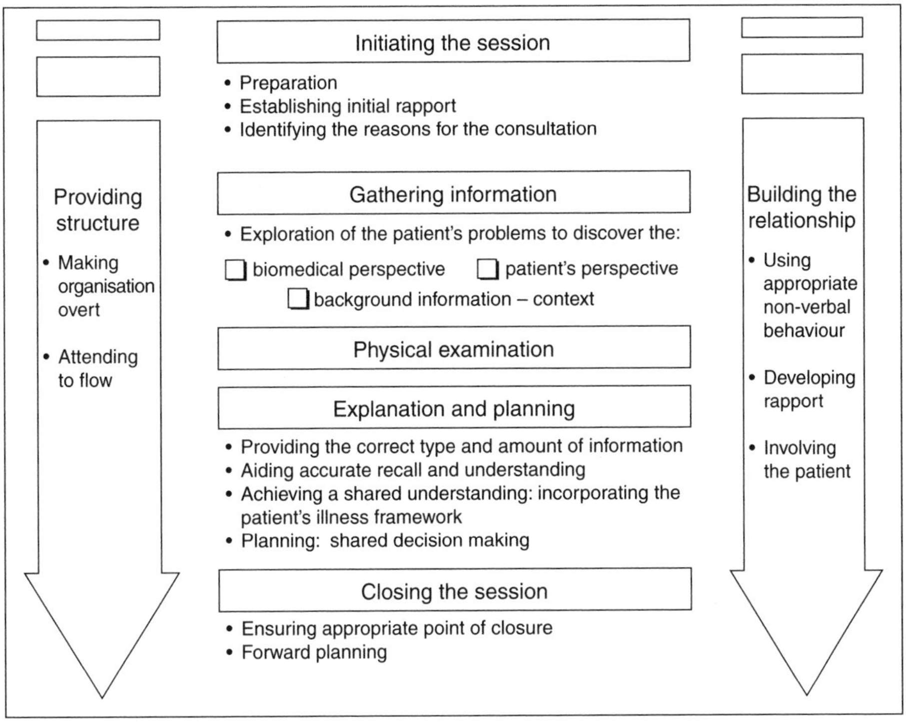

Providing structure

- Making organisation overt

- Attending to flow

Initiating the session

- Preparation
- Establishing initial rapport
- Identifying the reasons for the consultation

Gathering information

- Exploration of the patient's problems to discover the:

  ☐ biomedical perspective   ☐ patient's perspective
  ☐ background information – context

Physical examination

Explanation and planning

- Providing the correct type and amount of information
- Aiding accurate recall and understanding
- Achieving a shared understanding: incorporating the patient's illness framework
- Planning: shared decision making

Closing the session

- Ensuring appropriate point of closure
- Forward planning

Building the relationship

- Using appropriate non-verbal behaviour

- Developing rapport

- Involving the patient

Figure A2.2 Expanded framework.

Calgary–Cambridge Guide – communication process skills

Initiating the session

Establishing initial rapport

1 **Greets** patient and obtains patient's name
2 **Introduces** self, role and nature of interview; obtains consent if necessary
3 **Demonstrates respect** and interest; attends to patient's physical comfort

Identifying the reason(s) for the consultation

4 **Identifies** the patient's problems or the issues that the patient wishes to address with appropriate **opening question** (e.g. *'What problems brought you to the hospital?'* or *'What would you like to discuss today?'* or *'What questions did you hope to get answered today?'*)
5 **Listens** attentively to the patient's opening statement, without interrupting or directing patient's response
6 **Confirms list and screens** for further problems (e.g. *'So that's headaches and tiredness, anything else?'*)
7 **Negotiates agenda** taking both patient's and physician's needs into account

Gathering information

Exploration of patient's problems

8 **Encourages patient to tell the story** of the problem(s) from when first started to the present, in own words (clarifying reason for presenting now)
9 **Uses open and closed questioning techniques**, appropriately moving from open to closed
10 **Listens** attentively, allowing patient to complete statements without interruption and leaving space for patient to think before answering or go on after pausing
11 **Facilitates** patient's responses verbally and non-verbally, e.g. by use of encouragement, silence, repetition, paraphrasing, interpretation
12 **Picks up** verbal and non-verbal **cues** (body language, speech, facial expression); **checks out and acknowledges** as appropriate

13 **Clarifies** patient's statements that are unclear or need amplification (e.g. *'Could you explain what you mean by light-headed?'*)
14 Periodically **summarises** to verify own understanding of what the patient has said; invites patient to correct interpretation or provide further information
15 **Uses concise, easily understood questions and comments**; avoids or adequately explains jargon
16 **Establishes dates and sequence of events**

Additional skills for understanding the patient's perspective

17 **Actively determines and appropriately explores**:
   - patient's **ideas** (i.e. beliefs re cause)
   - patient's **concerns** (i.e. worries) regarding each problem
   - patient's **expectations**: (i.e. goals, what help the patient had expected for each problem)
   - **effects** – how each problem affects the patient's life
18 **Encourages patient to express feelings**

Providing structure to the consultation

Making organisation overt

19 **Summarises** at the end of a specific line of inquiry to confirm under-standing before moving on to the next section
20 **Progresses** from one section to another using **signposting, transitional statements**; includes rationale for next section

Attending to flow

21 Structures interview in logical **sequence**
22 Attends to **timing** and keeping interview on task

Building relationship

Using appropriate non-verbal behaviour

23 **Demonstrates appropriate non-verbal behaviour**:
   - eye contact, facial expression
   - posture, position, movement
   - vocal cues, e.g. rate, volume, intonation

24   If reads, writes **notes** or uses computer, does in a **manner that does not interfere with dialogue or rapport**

25   **Demonstrates** appropriate **confidence**

Developing rapport

26   **Accepts** legitimacy of patient's views and feelings; **is not judgemental**

27   **Uses empathy** to communicate understanding and appreciation of the patient's feelings or predicament; overtly **acknowledges patient's views and feelings**

28   **Provides support**: expresses concern, understanding, willingness to help; acknowledges coping efforts and appropriate self-care; offers partnership

29   **Deals sensitively** with embarrassing and disturbing topics and physical pain, including when associated with physical examination

Involving the patient

30   **Shares thinking** with patient to encourage patient's involvement (e.g. *'What I'm thinking now is . . .'*)

31   **Explains rationale** for questions or parts of physical examination that could appear to be non sequiturs

32   During **physical examination**, explains process, asks permission

Explanation and planning

Providing the correct amount and type of information

Aims: to give comprehensive and appropriate information
    to assess each individual patient's information needs
    to neither restrict nor overload

33   **Chunks and checks**: gives information in assimilable chunks; checks for understanding; uses patient's response as a guide to how to proceed

34   **Assesses patient's starting point**: asks for patient's prior knowledge early on when giving information; discovers extent of patient's wish for information

35   **Asks patient what other information would be helpful**, e.g. aetiology, prognosis

36   **Gives explanation at appropriate times**: avoids giving advice, information or reassurance prematurely

Aiding accurate recall and understanding

Aims: to make information easier for the patient to remember and understand

37 **Organises explanation**: divides into discrete sections; develops a logical sequence

38 **Uses explicit categorisation or signposting** (e.g. *'There are three important things that I would like to discuss. First . . .'; 'Now, shall we move on to . . .?'*)

39 **Uses repetition and summarising** to reinforce information

40 **Uses concise, easily understood language**; avoids or explains jargon

41 **Uses visual methods of conveying information**: diagrams, models, written information and instructions

42 **Checks patient's understanding** of information given (or plans made), e.g. by asking patient to restate in own words, clarifies as necessary

Achieving a shared understanding: incorporating the patient's perspective

Aims: to provide explanations and plans that relate to the patient's perspective

to discover the patient's thoughts and feelings about the information given

to encourage an interaction rather than one-way transmission

43 **Relates explanations to patient's perspective**: to previously elicited ideas, concerns and expectations

44 **Provides opportunities and encourages patient to contribute**: to ask questions, seek clarification or express doubts; responds appropriately

45 **Picks up and responds to verbal and non-verbal cues**, e.g. patient's need to contribute information or ask questions, information overload, distress

46 **Elicits patient's beliefs, reactions and feelings** re information given, terms used; acknowledges and addresses where necessary

Planning: shared decision making

Aims: to allow patient to understand the decision-making process

to involve patient in decision making to the level they wish

to increase patient's commitment to plans made

47 **Shares own thinking as appropriate**: ideas, thought processes and dilemmas

48 **Involves patient**:
   - offers suggestions and choices rather than directives
   - encourages patient to contribute their own ideas, suggestions

49 **Explores management options**
50 **Ascertains level of involvement patient wishes** in making the decision at hand
51 **Negotiates a mutually acceptable plan**:
   - signposts own position of equipoise or preference regarding available options
   - determines patient's preferences
52 **Checks with patient**:
   - if accepts plan
   - if concerns have been addressed

Closing the session

Forward planning

53 **Contracts** with patient re next steps for patient and physician
54 **Safety nets**, explaining possible unexpected outcomes, what to do if plan is not working, when and how to seek help

Ensuring appropriate point of closure

55 **Summarises** session briefly and clarifies plan of care
56 **Final check** that patient agrees and is comfortable with plan and asks if any corrections, questions or other issues

Options in explanation and planning (includes content and process skills)

If discussing opinion and significance of problem

57 Offers opinion of what is going on and names if possible
58 Reveals rationale for opinion
59 Explains causation, seriousness, expected outcome, short- and long-term consequences
60 Elicits patient's beliefs, reactions, concerns re opinion

If negotiating mutual plan of action

61 Discusses options, e.g. no action, investigation, medication or surgery, non-drug treatments (physiotherapy, walking aids, fluids, counselling), preventive measures

62 Provides information on action or treatment offered, names steps involved, how it works, benefits and advantages, possible side-effects

63 Obtains patient's view of need for action, perceived benefits, barriers, motivation

64 Accepts patient's views; advocates alternative viewpoint as necessary

65 Elicits patient's reactions and concerns about plans and treatments, including acceptability

66 Takes patient's lifestyle, beliefs, cultural background and abilities into consideration

67 Encourages patient to be involved in implementing plans, to take responsibility and be self-reliant

68 Asks about patient support systems; discusses other support available

If discussing investigations and procedures

69 Provides clear information on procedures, e.g. what patient might experience, how patient will be informed of results

70 Relates procedures to treatment plan: value, purpose

71 Encourages questions about and discussion of potential anxieties or negative outcomes

---

Reproduced with permission from Silverman J, Kurtz S, Draper J (2005) *Skills for Communicating with Patients* (2e). Radcliffe Publishing, Oxford.

Appendix III: Further reading

In this appendix, I offer a minimal but extremely high-quality list of further reading – from these volumes, the reader will be able to access the whole literature on doctor–patient communication. In particular, Silverman *et al.* and Tate offer extensive reading lists.

For medical students

This book is an excellent place to start reading about communication in medicine – if you want further reading, try Silverman *et al.*

- Lloyd M, Bor R (2004) *Communication Skills for Medicine* (2e). Churchill Livingstone, Edinburgh.

For doctors

These two books are complementary. Silverman *et al.* authoritatively review the current literature and present the Calgary–Cambridge Guide, an evidence-based approach to the core skills of doctor–patient communication. Tate offers a more conversational style from general practice, which is of particular relevance to GP registrars.

- Silverman J, Kurtz S, Draper J (2005) *Skills for Communicating with Patients* (2e). Radcliffe Publishing, Oxford.
- Tate P (2003) *The Doctor's Communication Handbook* (4e). Radcliffe Medical Press, Oxford.

For difficult communication

This book will raise the reader's awareness of further issues, such as communication with dying patients or using an interpreter.

- Macdonald E (ed.) (2004) *Difficult Conversations in Medicine*. Oxford University Press, Oxford.

Index

Page numbers in italics refer to figures.

'advanced access' arrangements   101–2
advocacy roles   62
anger in patients   54, 55–6
appointment length   35–6, 44, 76
   double sessions   96, 97–8
   long sessions   *101*
   patient choice   101–2
attachment theories   86–7
attendance frequency
   as cue   22
   see also frequent attendees
attitudes *see* doctor attitudes; patient's
      agenda; patient attitudes
availability   117
   see also work-home boundaries

Balint, M   5, 10, 85
Beckman, H and Frankel, R   24
bedside manners *see* communication skills
Bennet, G   144
bereavement
   and GP availability   117
   holding   70–1
   impact on GP   119, 121
   listening boundaries   38–9, 53–4, 70–1,
      119, 121
   long-term GP-patient relationships
      53–4, 70–1
Berger, P and Kellner, H   140
Blau, J   24
body language
   patient cues   22
   to discourage communication   *40*
   to promote interaction   23
boundaries   39–40, 105–14, 143–7
   and body language   *40*
   colleagues as patients   111–12
   friends as patients   109–11
   and location   112–13, 143–4, 146

organisational   96–8, 99–100
   patients as friends   106–9, 113–14
   terminal illness and bereavement   38–9,
      53–4, 70–1, 119, 121
   see also holding
Bowlby, J   86–7
Browne, K and Freeling, P   5, 88
Byrne, P and Long, B   5–6, 146–7

Calgary-Cambridge Guide (Silverman, Kurtz
      and Draper)   6, 162–9
Carey, G (Archbishop of Canterbury)   136
Choosing Talking Therapies? (DoH)   139
communication importance   140–2
communication skills   162–9
   information sources   170
   recognising cues   22–3
   use of silence   23–4
   see also consultation; listening; listening
      skills
computer use   99–100
*The Consultation: an approach to learning and
      teaching* (Pendleton *et al.*)   6
consultation
   factors impacting on encounters *130*
   frameworks and guides   6, *162–3*, 164–9
   as journey   131–2
   methods of analysis   6–7
   models   6–7
   pre- and post-modern technology   3–5
   pressures and stress   95–102, 105–6, 129
   tasks   6
   theory vs current restraints   10–11, 148,
      156
   as therapeutic encounter   4–5
   time and length issues   35–6, 44, 76,
      95–102
   see also doctor-patient relationships;
      holding; listening

consultation rates   97, 99–102
   longer sessions   *101*
continuity of care   135–6
counselling
   beyond GPs remit   77
   referrals from GPs   40–2, 62
   as role for GPs   138–40
crying with patients   145
cues   21–3
   defined   21
   non-verbal   22
   taxonomy   23
   types *22*

delegation   100
demanding patients   54–5, 82
   frequent attendees   88
   and holding   88–9
Department of Health, on 'talking
      therapies'   139
dependency   38, 55, 73–4, 81
   and holding   72–4, 79–81
   use of listening boundaries   38
   see also frequent attendees
depressive disorders, and holding   71–2
detachment   118–9
diagnosis, as problem-solving   124–5
difficult patients   54–5, 82, 84–5
   and holding   88–9
   and sincerity   129
   see also dependency
doctor attitudes, towards
   colleagues as patients   111–12
   counselling   41–2
   dependency   79–81
   diagnosis   60, 124–5
   difficult patients   54–6
   friend-patient boundaries   107–9,
      110–11, 113
   general practice   123–7
   GP-patient relations   49–52
   limiting listening   36–9
   listening skills   41–2
   long/double appointments   97
   own ill health   120
   own limitations   41–2, 125–7
   pastoral listening work   63–5
   present-giving   109

sincerity   127–9
value of listening   32, 97–8
work-life balance   115–17
workload   99–100
see also doctor-patient relationships
doctor-patient encounters *see* consultation;
      doctor-patient relationships
doctor-patient relationships   49–57
   attachment theories   86–7
   colleagues as patients   111–12
   and continuity   135–6
   detachment and personal
         boundaries   118–19
   friends as patients   109–11
   'important' patients   52
   influencing factors   37, 49–50
   interpersonal boundaries   105–14,
      143–7
   involvement and significance   49–52
   key difficulties   54–6
   long-term associations   52–4
   over dependency   38, 55, 73–4
   paternalistic vs. patient empowered   65
   and patient satisfaction   42–3
   patients as friends   106–9
   power issues   142–7
   trust and respect   50, 55, 64–5, 85–6
   see also holding
The Doctor, His Patient and The Illness
      (Balint)   5
The Doctor's Communication Handbook
      (Tate)   170
doctors
   behaviour patterns   5–6
   comparisons with hospital doctors   5
   counsellor/support role studies   138
   as patients   111–12, 120, 144–5
   as performers   128–9, 145, 147
   self-awareness through work   119–22
   see also doctor attitudes; doctor-patient
      relationships; workload
*Doctors Talking to Patients: a study of the
      verbal behaviour of general practitioners in
      their surgeries* (Byrne and Long)
      5–6
double appointments   96, 97–8
Dowrick, C   142
'the drug doctor' (Balint)   10

E4 model (Keller and Carroll)   6
ego-support   87
emotional stress, and interpersonal
      boundaries   105–6, 145
enabling relationships   89–90
encounter
   defined   x
   types   134–5
   see also consultation; doctor-patient
      relationships
*European Definition of General Practice/Family
      Medicine*   9
   and pastoral work   138

family life, impact on work   120–1
Five conceptual dimensions for patient-
      centredness (Mead and Bower)   9–10
Fleischman, Paul   141
A Fortunate Man (Sassall)   141–2
frequent attendees
   defined   88
   see also dependency
Freud, S   136
friends, as patients   109–11
Fry, John   138
Fugelli, P   135

general practice
   definitions and characteristics   9
   management of workloads   97–8, 99
   optimal size   101
   as separate discipline   4
   technology and computer use
      99–100
   and 'therapeutical relationship'
      development (Balint)   4–5
Gibson, R   3–4
gifts   56, 109
Gore, J and Ogden, J   43
GPs
   behaviour patterns   5–6
   comparisons with hospital doctors   5
   counsellor/support role studies   138
   as patients   111–12, 120, 144–5
   as performers   128–9, 145, 147
   self-awareness through work   119–22
   see also doctor attitudes; doctor-patient
      relationships; workload

health, and stress   84
'heartsink' patients   55, 82, 84–5
   holding   88–9
   and sincerity   129
holding
   attachment theory   86–7
   definitions and key issues   137
   descriptions and examples   67–8
   and difficult patients   88–9
   GP's self-perception   83–4
   'listening as work' model   133, 135
   mental health problems   70, 71–2, 138
   methods and management   72–4
   over-dependency   79–81, 88–9
   patient-centredness   89–90
   problems and inappropriate support
      74–8
   rationale   70–2
   and trust   85–6
   types   68–70
   value and significance   81–5
home life   115–16
   see also work-home boundaries
home visits   100
   over-demanding patients   56
Howie, J *et al.*   89

interaction, defined ix
involvement   49–52
   and significance   51–2

Jung, C   136

Kalamazoo consensus statement   7

Lang, F *et al.*   23
Levinson, W *et al.*   21
life events, and holding   71
listening
   and choice   29–33
   as GP role   59–60
   'here and now' vs. over time   10
   limiting factors   35–9
   sharing and referring   40–2
   significance for patients   17–20, 33
   time pressures   35–6
   see also cues; pastoral listening work

'listening loops'   29–33, 132
    defined   32
    diagrammatic representation   30
listening skills
    body language   23
    cues   21–3
    limiting/blocking methods   39–40
    models for practice   29–33, 132–5
    recognising cues   20–5, 29–32
    recognising patient agendas   20–5
    use of silence   23–4
    see also pastoral listening work
'listening as work' model   132–5
    and continuity of care   135–6
    diagrammatic representation   133
    and holding   135
    levels   133–4
    and pastoral work   132
locum doctors   100
long-term relationships   52–4
    see also holding

McKevitt, C and Morgan, M   144
marital and relationship problems   71
May, C et al.   146
Mead, N and Bower, P   9–10, 89
Mechanic, D and Meyer, S   85–6
mental health problems, and holding   70,
    71–2, 138
micro-analysis (consultation)   6–7
Miller, W   134–5
models for consultations   6–7
    technical representations   6–7
    whole person/long-term approaches
        7–8
models of GP-patient encounter   131
models for listening
    'listening loops'   29–33, 30, 132
    'listening as work'   133, 132–5

narrative medicine   1–3
    and story-telling   2
The Nature of General Medical Practice
    (RCGP)   9
Neighbour, R   6, 21, 32, 118, 131
new patients   21
Nicholls, L   3
non-verbal cues
    of patient's agenda   22

    to discourage communication   40
    to promote interaction   23–4

pastoral listening work   59–65, 137–40
    definitions and key issues   137
    descriptions and examples   60–2
    difficulties   64–5
    doctor attitudes   63–5
    'listening as work' model   132, 133
patient satisfaction studies   42–3
patient-centredness   147–8
    as model for consultation   7–8
    Five conceptual dimensions (Mead and
        Bower)   9–10
    and holding   89–90
    and pragmatism   11
patient's agenda
    changing GPs   54
    desire for friendship   107–9,
        113–14
    non-verbal cues   24–5
    prioritising 'lists'   95–6
    sensitive topics   43
patient attitudes
    anger and animosity   55–6
    on choice of GP   42–3
    friendliness   106–9
    on GP practice and approaches
        9, 10
patient's story, relevance   1–2
Pendleton, D et al.   6
power issues   142–3
    and boundaries   143–7
    person-person encounters   145–6
present-giving   56, 109
process analysis, in consultation   6–7
professionalism, confidence and trust   55,
    64–5

RCGP (Royal College of General
    Practitioners)
    on the nature of general practice   9
    on technical/pastoral balance   137
relationship, defined   ix
religion
    GPs as 'the new clergy'   136–7
    and sincerity   128–9
    see also pastoral listening work

Sassall, John   141–2
self-awareness   119–22
  factors impacting on encounters   *130*
  and power issues   146–7
self-doubts   125–7
sexual behaviours   56
shared decision-making   10
shared listening   40–2, 62
silence, listening skills   23–4
Silverman, J, Kurtz, S and Draper, J   6,
    162–70
six-component patient-centred model
    (Stewart *et al.*) 7–8
Skills for Communicating with Patients
    (Silverman *et al.*)   162–9
Snow, R   136
social functions   136–7
  see also pastoral listening work
Stewart, M *et al.*   7–8, 147
story telling   2–3
stress
  effects on patient health   84
  from patient encounters   105–6
  on GPs   95, 105–6
  and maintaining sincerity   129
study
  aims   ix
  methodology   161
  terminology   ix–x

Tate, P   170
telephone availability   116–17
terminal illness
  and GP availability   117
  and GP-patient relationships   53–4

impact on GP   119, 121
and listening boundaries   38–9
The Doctor-Patient Relationship (Browne and
    Freeling)   5
therapeutic alliance   9–10
Three Function Approach (Cohen-Cole)   6
time pressures   95–102
  coping skills   100
  and GP stress   95
  impact on listening   35–6, 44
  prioritising patient problems   95–6
  prioritising patients   96–8
  and running late   99
  technology and computer use   99–100
  see also appointment length; workload
Tonge, W   21
trust   50
  in GP as 'professional'   55, 64–5
  and holding   85–6
Tuckett, D *et al.*   10

Williams, M and Neal, R   101
Winnicott, D   87
'witnessed significance' (Fleischman)   141
work-home boundaries   115–22
  living locally   116–17
  patient transgressions   112–13
  taking work home   115–16
  telephone availability   116–17
workload
  and consultation length   76, 97–8
  management and equal distribution
    97–8
  non-surgery factors   100
  prioritising patients   96–8
  structural pressures   98–102